Feed Your Body Right

To Maribelle Davis
I thank you for
a wonderful Evening!

Lendall Small

27 mar 96

Feed Your Body Right

UNDERSTANDING YOUR INDIVIDUAL BODY CHEMISTRY FOR PROPER NUTRITION WITHOUT GUESSWORK

Dr. Smith's unique plan to help the sick, the tired, the weak, the sad, the heavy, and the discouraged. New—but really old—ways to treat old and new problems. Any procedure that does not include a strict accounting of an individual's body chemistry does not meet basic chemical laws by which we all operate. The program described in the book should clearly and logically lead you to vibrant health.

LENDON H. SMITH, M.D.

M. Evans and Company, Inc.
New York

M. Evans and Company, Inc.
216 East 49th Street
New York, New York 10017

Library of Congress Cataloging-in-Publication Data

Smith, Lendon H., 1921–
    Feed your body right : understanding your individual body chemistry : choosing your dietary supplements without guesswork / by Lendon H. Smith.
      p.   cm.
    Includes bibliographical references and index.
    ISBN 0-87131-776-1 : $12.95
    1. Nutrition. 2. Health. 3. Body composition. 4. Nutritionally induced diseases. I. Title.
RA784.S59   1993
613.2—dc20
                              93-41969
                                 CIP

Manufactured in the United States of America
Typeset by AeroType, Inc.

9 8 7 6 5 4 3 2 1

Dedication

This book is dedicated to my dear wife, Julie, and my patients, who knew that I was up to something and had the patience and tact to let me try a few things out (on them).

Thanks to John Kitkoski, a chemistry genius, who has given me the insights and the knowledge that I needed to write this book. He showed me that chemistry is basic to everything we are and do.

I am indebted to the naturopathic physicians who have shown me that there are better ways to solve health problems than just throwing drugs at the sick. They know that if the territory (the body) is healthy, germs, viruses, and stressors cannot hurt humans. Glen Nagel, N.D., was especially helpful with the section on herbs. Dick Thom, N.D., D.D.S., gave me insights about food sensitivities.

A Note from Dr. Richard Marsh

In February 1992, I stepped off the plane at Portland, Oregon, to be greeted by Dr. Lendon Smith—a man I had been told I just had to meet. For some seventeen years I had been in practice as a family physician, and I had become jaded with the traditional and often ineffective approach to illness—diagnosis, treatment with heavy reliance on pharmaceuticals, little or no emphasis on prevention or diet. Over the years I had learned how to treat using diets and nutritional supplements but real success seemed to be eluding me as I stumbled along using empirical methods. Finally I had won a traveling fellowship to study nutritional medicine in the United States.

Here I was meeting a complete stranger who had kindly invited me to stay with him with the words, "We in the States know everything and welcome any naive British types who might help us spread the word!"

Lendon introduced me to many exciting new people and ideas but best of all he introduced me to the Life Balances Health Program. New, novel, simple but precise and effective it has subtly altered my career. The Life Balances Health Program has changed his, and my, approach to medicine and the treatment of patients. This book shows what it is all about.

Dr. Richard Marsh
Buckingham, England

Contents

Preface

We all want to be as healthy as possible. We want advice about our health. We know that if we are healthy we will feel good and be cheerful, and will be able to handle most of life's stressors. If we feel sick, we go to a doctor hoping that it is only a minor problem and it can easily and painlessly be corrected—and not cost much. We want advice about diet, and what supplements we should take to avoid getting sick. Most of us would rather save the use of drugs until we are hit with some "nasty" like pneumonia or for the temporary relief of insomnia or the control of allergies. Some of us even seek drugless methods of disease control, through naturopathic medicine, homeopathy, or chiropractic adjustments to get rid of our uncomfortable symptoms. And some of us even ask the doctors, "Why did I get sick?"

The standard allopathic doctors (M.D.s) may not be able to answer that last query except to say, "Stress," and then shrug their shoulders. They are trained to make a positive diagnosis of an identifiable disease and then prescribe the appropriate drug or offer the indicated surgery. The detective work of discovering the diagnosis is the basic tenet (and fun) of medical practice. They received this training in medical school, and it is reenforced when they attend medical conferences and read medical literature. The pharmaceutical industry appears to "own" the doctors' medical journals and consequently the doctors' minds. And they still do not answer the patients' question, "Why did I get sick?"

I am going to provide you with an answer to that question by introducing you to a program that will help you feel better, reduce your perception of stress, and eliminate symptoms and signs that suggest deviations from health. If you have a *bona fide* diagnosed disease, this program should allow you to obtain a state of health that is incompatible with that disease.

This program is based on solid chemical laws so its scientific basis cannot be disputed. (If a person has asthma and his calcium level in his blood is low, and then, if he gets calcium, and his asthma disappears, his asthma was due to a low calcium level.)

This book will instruct you about the metabolic workings of your body. You will become more accountable for your own health. Your senses of smell and taste will guide you in your choices of supplements—it is that simple. The computer analysis of your blood test results will indicate what you need on day one, then your nose and tongue will guide your food and nutrient choices after that. This program makes allowances for your individual differences due to your genetics and the foods you choose to eat.

You can and should be responsible for your own health. Your health care provider will then be able to take a secondary—but important—teacher role.

Any symptom you have—fatigue, obesity, allergies, aches, depression—can be traced back to some tilt in your chemistry. Chemistry is basic to the function of the enzymes of the body. If the concentrations and the ratios of those elements are not exactly right for your body's functions you will develop symptoms. It is your body's way to tell you that something is wrong and to motivate you to do something about it.

Genetics play a role in most conditions of the flesh. While genes may not determine everything about you, they will make you more susceptible to a wide range of such conditions as obesity, hypertension, diabetes, arthritis, alcoholism, enuresis, hyperactivity, and even influence such personality traits as shyness, extroversion, and depression. At least we have moved away from the concept that if we do not quite understand the origin of a condition, it must be psychogenic.

This book will give you new ways of understanding your nutritional needs and preferences. Your mother may have told you to eat your vegetables, but maybe vegetables didn't taste good to you. (Perhaps she boiled everything to death.) Now you eat them because you are trying to motivate your children, or because your doctor said you had to. But the reason you did not like what your mother served you was that your biochemical system was crying out for *acidic* foods while she continued to serve you *alkaline* ones. At the present time most of us in North America are somewhat alkaline, and our metabolic needs encourage us to eat acidic foods. There are reasons like this one behind most food preferences. Often, food preferences, food allergies, over-weight—a whole range of nutritional problems—are linked direct-ly to a person's specific nutritional requirements. Understanding your personal nutritional makeup can help you follow a logical, unique, personalized diet that will lead you to better health. This book will show you how.

If you can understand a few basic chemical rules about how your body works, you will be your own guide to achieving health. You will need your health provider less and less. You will be free from symptoms and you may even develop a buoyancy and a zest for life.

The key principle behind my book is: no more guesswork.

1

"Why Do I Get Sick?"

Today most people know there is a nutritional or biochemical basis for many diseases. They expect their doctors to discover the triggering event of the sickness and then guide them to a healthier lifestyle to reverse the disease or at least prevent its recurrence. Because many doctors fail to teach their patients the methods for correcting diet and lifestyle, people often resort to self-help books. If you are one of the millions of people who has tried, repeatedly and unsuccessfully, to lose weight, to feel better, to be healthier, or to have more energy based on a "scheme"—I have good news that will delight you because it is simple, precise, scientifically accurate, and medically sound. What you are about to read will give you a radically new way of looking at your problems and, what's more, the means to overcome them.

Your Unique Chemistry

The reason your regime failed was that it didn't take into account your body's chemistry. People think it absurd if I suggest they buy a generic dress or move into a generic house, but are perfectly willing to follow a generic diet plan that doesn't take into account the specific needs of their unique chemistry. What you need—and what I can give you—is an individualized system, one that is tailored for you and your body, and wonder of wonders, based on the universal, chemical laws of the universe, which we all obey.

Each of us is unique, like a snowflake. Therefore, no one, not even a nutritionist, can prescribe what you should eat, what exercise program is best for you, and what lifestyle you should adopt without first asking a few questions about you and your lineage. With just a little genetic information (family susceptibilities), some blood studies, a measure of the pulse rate and the blood pressure, an individualized nutritional program can be planned that will work for your particular body type and metabolism. You can do some of this yourself.

I began my career as a pediatrician. In the last twenty-five years, I've moved progressively away from a traditional medical practice and turned more and more toward nutrition as the solution to many of my patients' ills. Some years ago I perceived the connection between nutrition and health problems because of personal experiences. One of my children was a bed wetter and another was hyperactive. The conventional, psychiatric approach toward bed-wetting claims that the cause is an emotional problem: The child hates the mother and is paying her back for some real or imagined hurt by wetting the bed. Treatment consists of attempting to substitute oral aggression for urethral hostility. Get the child to verbalize his anger.

This didn't make much sense to my wife. "Our son doesn't wet every night. Doesn't he hate me every day?" When we realized that he only wet on those nights when he'd drunk milk during the day, we stopped giving him dairy products and the problem disappeared. It was as easy as that.

One daughter had a problem settling down in school. "She's not working up to her potential," we'd hear. "She has good and bad days . . . is distracted . . . could do better if she would try harder . . ." We used the standard stimulant medication prescribed for hyperactivity for a year or so until we found that cutting down on sugar and getting her to eat more frequently helped her concentration and attention span. Even today she must snack every two to three hours to keep herself on an even keel.

Genetics Explains Some Diseases

I was positive that genetic factors were involved in both these conditions. In the first case, I, myself, had been a bed wetter and my son is practically my clone physically. When I confessed my childhood secret to my wife, she said I should have told her about this *before* we were married. "Bad traits come from the father's side of the family," she observed. However, I felt obliged to point out to her that we both shared some of our daughter's traits. Somewhat reluctantly she had to agree.

But though fate may have handed you some negative genetic traits, many of them may be offset. While genes determine your susceptibility to certain diseases, it is clear that such diseases need not become manifest unless your lifestyle—including several factors, chiefly diet—allows them to surface. Changing your lifestyle could preclude your particular family disease from appearing or, at least, could minimize its effects.

Becoming aware of the link between genetic predisposition and the role of diet was an important breakthrough for me. I discovered I could determine, and sometimes predict, the course of an illness when I made such a connection.

My son's medical history was a perfect example: a genetic weakness made manifest by a dietary insult. Even if we boiled the cow's milk for four hours, he suffered from colic. When he was a year old, milk gave him ear infections; at two, it gave him asthma. Then came the bed-wetting, followed in adolescence by headaches, phlegm, and acne. As an adult he would become constipated or develop a rash on his buttocks if he drank milk. By reacting to dairy products with all these symptoms, it appeared as if the body was trying to get its owner's attention: "Yoo hoo! If you don't get the message that milk is giving you an earache or sinus trouble, how would you like a migraine, a bloody nose, or a boil?"

Often, if my patients' parents were obese, hyperactive, alcoholic, or diabetic, I noted that these kids were more likely to be sugar-holics, overweight, or hyperactive. If sugar, preservatives, additives, and empty-calorie foods were not held in check, these children were unable to concentrate or would be overwhelmed with mood swings. If the amount was controlled—provided the parents changed their children's diets—the symptoms disappeared.

True, this dietary management didn't work on everyone. However, it did work often enough—in 60 percent of cases—that I was convinced that regulation of diet was a valid concept and a first step in controlling these problems.

In treating hyperactive kids nutritionally, I quickly found out that it was next to impossible to get them to change their diet without dealing with the diet of the entire family. Just try to get a child to be satisfied with a carrot (a CARROT? or an APPLE?) for dessert when the rest of the family is having cherry pie à la mode!

Most of the parents who carefully followed the suggested regime would return in three weeks with the delightful news that not only were their kids "better" (calmer, more cheerful, and more attentive) but—wonder of wonders—they, who were both overweight, were losing weight, as much as two pounds a week.

I, too, was delighted. I had apparently discovered a cure-all diet. So I began to try a no-sugar, no-junk food, limited-dairy diet on anyone who walked into the office. But although it worked in many cases, it did not in all. I worked with chiropractors, naturopathic physicians, acupuncturists, nutritionists, and kinesiologists and discovered that even though a treatment works on one patient, it will not necessarily work on the next patient with identical complaints.

After a bit of research on my part, I realized I had not accounted for some very important factors such as body type, glandular function, or individual biochemistries.

2

How I Got from There to Here

Call it science. Call it the state of the art of medicine. I now believe what I learned in medical school in the early 1940s was a calculated effort by the pharmaceutical industry to get fledgling medical doctors to use drugs, their drugs.

Drugs, Drugs, Drugs

We were taught to make a diagnosis, clear and simple. Once a label was attached to the patient, a drug was attached to the disease label. It was neat and clean. If we could not remember the name of the drug, the pharmaceutical representative (drug rep) who came to our offices once or twice a month reminded us. Ads in the medical journals kept the name alive in our memory storage banks.

Pneumonia? Strep throat? Think of penicillin. Kidney or bladder infection? Try the new sulfa drug. During the Second World War sulfa powder was sprinkled into open wounds and the peritoneal cavity to suppress infection. (All the German soldiers in Italy were given a sulfa drug prophylactically to preclude wound infections. By the time the American and British soldiers got there the Italian women had developed a very resistant form of gonorrhea.)

Seizure disorders were partially controlled with sedative drugs. Adrenal gland-stimulating drugs were synthesized in the early 1940s, and then the manufacturing and marketing of other human hormones followed. Many of these were found to be lifesaving for asthmatics and those with autoimmune diseases.

Surgery became innovative. Congenital malformations such as cleft palate, heart lesions, and musculo-skeletal anomalies could be corrected. Hernias and congenital bowel obstructions were fixed routinely. Tumors once believed to be too remote for removal were accessible with the new techniques.

Diagnostic laboratory testing became efficient. Enzyme levels in the blood indicated a liver disease or a suspected heart attack. The thyroid gland function could be assayed more accurately than by relying on the old breathing test. Doctors thought that with only two teaspoonfuls of blood from the patient, a history or physical examination was unnecessary—the diagnosis was clearly in the lab results.

When I started practice drugs were instantly available by prescription. Drugstores were well stocked and ready to supply a pharmaceutical for almost every disease that surfaced.

It was fun. I was an expert. People came to me for the latest in science, and I had it. Unfortunately, we had nothing for the viruses until a secondary bacterial infection set in, but then we could prescribe an antibiotic.

But at no time did we receive—either in lectures or journal articles—any clue of how or why our patients got sick in the first place.

Does someone get TB because he was inhaling when a contagious TB sufferer was exhaling? Why does one child get but ten chicken pox sores and her sibling get one hundred of them plus ulcers in his throat and a high fever? Why do Japanese–American women have a higher rate of breast cancer than their sisters in Japan?

Where are the answers?

John Kitkoski Appears

Almost ten years ago, John Kitkoski, a man from Spokane, called me. He said, "Dr. Smith, I believe I can make you more credible with your listeners, and at the same time you might be able to help us with our program." He continued: "I have been working with animals for twenty-five years and now I have designed a program for humans. I have studied animal husbandry, soil agronomy, chemistry, and biochemistry. By putting all these things together I realized that human function is based on the immutable laws of chemistry."

SENSE OF SMELL IS HOOKED UP WITH THE BRAIN

He told me about his horses. He studied the chemicals in their blood. Some of them were low in calcium, some low in magnesium, and some in zinc. He mixed extra calcium in one of the food troughs, some magnesium in another, and some zinc in a third. The animals smelled each of the troughs. The horses that were low in calcium only ate from the calcium-supplemented feed. The animals low in magnesium, ate from the magnesium-supplemented feed, and the same with the low-zinc ones. He said, "That is why the nose is in front of the mouth, and not in your armpit." When the horses moved away from the nutrient-supplemented feed and back to the standard feed, he checked the mineral levels in their blood and found out that the blood levels had moved close to the normal range. Their senses of smell told them when and how much they needed.

Then he asked, "Dr. Smith, do you know why a lactating cow will never eat grass that has ever had manure on it?"

"That makes sense to me. I wouldn't eat it either."

He explained that manure makes the soil and the grass growing from it alkaline, and the small brain of the cow senses that the calcium in the milk she will produce will be too alkaline to be soluble, and will not get through the lacteals in her udder. A caked breast is very painful in all lactating mammals.

He then explained why a pregnant woman, when she's about six months along, will send her husband out in the middle of the night for some ice cream and pickles; ice cream for the calcium, and pickles to acidify the calcium. The baby will not get the calcium for his rapidly growing bones unless it is in an acid medium. Kitkoski made enough sense that I got involved with his program. I have used it on my family, myself, and have encouraged people to try it.

The senses of smell and taste are there to protect us from the environment's toxins. Our sense of smell is where it is to tell us what is good or bad for our body. The nose is not in the armpit nor the groin; it is in front of the mouth to help monitor what is about to be put into the body. It also tells us if a food is good enough to eat. The sense of taste is the next line of protection for the body. If something tastes bad, it will be spat out.

Kitkoski pointed out that the cells of the olfactory and gustatory sense organs are connected to the brain. The brain is bathed in the blood from the rest of the body. Receptive cells there act like electron probes to signal what is needed. The brain can detect whether a nutrient is worth pursuing. If the blood is low in something that is detected by the sense of smell, it signals the brain, which then sets up foraging activity to get the item, eat it, and swallow it. The body needed it at that time. For example, if you are thirsty, the cells of the hypothalmus in the lower brain are dehydrated as well as the cells in the rest of the body. These special cells signal the cortex of the brain to find some water. When the right amount of water has been swallowed, the cells are hydrated within seconds, and the satisfied cells tell the cortex to signal the owner to put the glass of water down.

I joined up with Kitkoski and his program ten years ago. Since then I have not been disappointed. I was confused in the beginning because this method of controlling disease was so different from my medical training based on the paradigm: Make a diagnosis and prescribe a remedy. The Life Balances Health Program does not rely upon a diagnosis or a label. The program makes people accountable for their own health by showing them how to follow explicit, immutable chemical laws.

To make this transition as linear as possible, I must make a medical journey through time.

3

A Very Brief History of Mankind's Efforts to Improve Health

Hippocrates

Every Western approach to medical history begins with a summary of Hippocrates's life. Born in 460 B.C., Hippocrates was a pioneer. He was renowned for his accurate observations. He believed that diseases were the result of natural causes. Therefore, nature was the healer, but the patient was to be an active participant. Imbalances of the four humours (blood, phlegm, yellow bile, black bile) explained the disease condition, and these were affected by seasons and diet. "Let your medicine be your food, and your food be your medicine," is his most famous quote. Along with diet changes, he prescribed rest, washing, sympathy, and encouragement.

Acupuncture and Ayurvedic Medicines

The Orientals were using acupuncture as far back as 4,000 B.C. with success. Ayurvedic medicine started up about the same time in India and is still popular there. Each area had its medical practitioners, and codified systems of healing. Most of the world's populations used local plants, teas, extracts, and poultices, but the knowledge was transferred orally and some medical methods have been lost.

Galen

Galen, born in 130 A.D., was trained by the best authorities of the time. He was born a Greek but moved to Rome. He washed the wounds of the gladiators with red wine and saved many of these men from fatal infections. But, because he could not find better ways of explaining illnesses—other than the humours that were popular with the ancients before him—his antiquated ideas prevailed for centuries, and thus stifled medical progress. He did believe, however, that some weakness of the patient allowed sickness to invade.

Paracelsus

Paracelsus, born in Switzerland in 1493, used what he had learned from his patients and so broke from Galen's dogma. He traveled and gathered information from barber-surgeons, midwives, old wives, and whomever was the local healer. It was an empirical approach. He felt nature should heal wounds, but he did introduce mercury, sulfur, lead, gold, and even arsenic to the therapeutic armamentarium. Some of his treatments ended up as cures. He felt humans were governed by the environment and that doctors must study chemistry. He believed that all humans are imbued with a vital force and if that becomes weakened, disease will surely follow.

Cures were rare in those dead days. Survival was possible despite the "treatments." The healers were working in the dark. They had minimal knowledge of anatomy, physiology, and biochemistry. (Average life span was only about 20 to 30 years anyway.)

Lind

James Lind in the 18th century was instrumental in helping the British government see the value of citrus fruits in preventing scurvy in sailors on their long sailing trips. It only took about fifty years or so to convince the authorities it would save lives!

Pasteur

Louis Pasteur, born in 1822, had to battle the doctors who were steadfast in their belief in the dogma of the mid-19th century. When he discovered the bacteria that were associated with diseases, he felt the virulence of germs was the critical factor. He finally admitted on his deathbed that it was the territory (the body) that, when weakened, allowed the germs to invade.

Over the centuries these local efforts became codified into systems of healing. People used what was available, as they had no other choices. With commerce and communication peoples exchanged therapies. The colonists brought the "wonders" of European medicine with them: bloodletting, mercury salts, arsenic, and some herbs. They also learned therapies from the Native Americans. Priessnitz had discovered the value of hydrotherapy in Austria in the early 19th century. Sam Hahnemann founded the homeopathic method of like cures like. One hundred years ago 30 percent of medical doctors were using homeopathy in their practice. It was also about then that the pioneer American chiropractor, Daniel D. Palmer (1845–1913) realized that the flow of nerve energy could be freed by spinal manipulation.

Only a few of us were around eighty years ago when life was simpler. People then had to work physically hard. Farming, fishing, lumbering, ranching, washing, sewing, cooking, and building were the main occupations. Some diseases took a huge toll. If you got sick with one of the nasty ones, you died. Pneumonia, tuberculosis, typhoid fever, abscesses, osteomyelitis, meningitis, scarlet fever, peritonitis, erysipelas, childbed fever—all the bacterial infections were rampant in those days. Hospitals with their aspirin, purges, baths, and mercury treatments were ineffective in curing these overwhelming infections.

Addiction

In 1912 a higher percentage of people were addicted to morphine than at any other time in American history. It was used in most cough syrups, because it was the most effective cough suppressant. The cough might disappear, but the addiction continued.

The Harrison Narcotic Act of 1912 put a damper on morphine's use.

We had our Typhoid Mary, the 1918–19 influenza epidemic, and the streptococcus that was passed on to the public by the milk handlers. A cleaner life plus some prudent hand washing improved the health of the nation—or at least controlled some bacterial infections.

Degenerative diseases were almost unheard of partly because people were dying of other things before they got old enough to be in the age group to *acquire* a degenerative disease. Cancer was around, but not at today's rates. Heart attacks were rare. High blood pressure was present but did not lead to the rate of strokes that we see now. Those who did live to a ripe old age had somehow missed the fatal infections. Most of them were stiff, sore, and moved slowly, but they were alive and their long-term memory was intact.

The health advice in those early days of the 20th century had our grandparents believing that we must sleep with the windows open, drink three glasses of pure spring water daily, walk in the fresh air for thirty minutes daily, keep the bowels open, and have no negative thoughts. (Dancing, however, was thought to produce pelvic congestion and increase the risk of sterility for both male and female!)

In the second decade of this century the members of the American Medical Association decided that they alone were privy to the scientific basis of medical practice. They wisely eliminated some of the medical diploma mills of the time and laid down a rigorous curriculum aimed at teaching medical aspirants the "science" of medicine. Better microscopes, laboratory analyses, and X-ray diagnoses allowed the doctors to become better clinicians, but they still could not heal the really sick unless the infection localized itself to a boil with "laudable pus." It seemed a natural progression of logic to blame bacteria for disease; the "territory" was not important. It was the pathogen. They could now see the little bugs.

Antibiotics

In the nick of time, antibiotics arrived in the 1930s and 1940s. Then these allopaths *knew* they were on the real route to medical truth. But in the fifty years since then the dream of the final answer to infectious disease has become a nightmare. Modern medicine, based on the paradigm of find-the-germ-and-kill-it, put all its emphasis on this one battle, but they lost the war. It was exciting to see near-death pneumonia patients come to life with intravenous penicillin, but medical teaching failed to address the problem of why the person (territory) got sick in the first place.

Dad

My father was a pediatrician. He was modern, scientific, and respected by his peers. Get this for science in the 1920s to the late 1930s: It was standard medical practice in his day to fluoroscope babies to search for the enlarged thymus, which "everyone knew" was the cause of Sudden Infant Death Syndrome (SIDS), as a large thymus would crush the windpipe. If you did not have a fluoroscope, you were a bad doctor. "It is standard medical practice," is how the fluoroscope salesman got Dad to buy one. Then if Dad found an enlarged thymus in one of those little infants, he sent that baby off to a radiologist who x-rayed the gland down to a more "normal" size. It was almost an emergency to get this done before the thymus suffocated the child!

Dad was always supposed to wear the lead gloves, but sometimes he forgot. After twenty years he developed cancer of his fingers, and six of them had to be amputated, and skin grafts were necessary for the rest. Some of the children who had their thymuses irradiated grew up to develop cancer of the thyroid. That was science in the '20s and '30s. One wonders what we are doing now that will be an embarrassment to the medical profession in the years to come.

Some progress has been made on the way to universal health, but it does not seem to me to have anything to do with the miracles of "modern" medicine. We are still at the mercy of impoverished top soil, toxic air and water, and the inappropriate remedies from the pharmaceutical industry.

I believe we must junk much of the prescription approach to modern treatment and get back to a cleaner lifestyle of fresh fruits and vegetables, low-fat protein, and whole grains. We have the germs under some control, now we have to improve the immune system of the population and help calm the stresses of life that lead to allergies and virus infections.

(I don't think we should cut out the dancing, however. Dancing might lead to fecundity, but it will not affect fertility.)

If you take a few vitamins and minerals and make a visit to your friendly chiropractor or naturopathic physician, you will get to feeling better, and that makes sense to me. However, it may not be enough.

If modern medicine saves lives, why are we as a nation so unhealthy? And for all the good that these drugs do, why are they so costly and dangerous? We do need the biotechnology, but we have to revive the almost forgotten, time-honored, natural, drug-less methods of nutrition, botanical medicine, Chinese herbs, acupuncture, homeopathy, physical medicine, and even vibra-tional therapies plus the approaches afforded by psychospiritual methods.

Allopathic medicine is "modern" medicine. Make a diagnosis, and cure the disease with drugs. One definition is "produce a condition in the body incompatible with the disease." If you have enough penicillin in you, you will not have a strep throat. By the same token, if you can improve the power of the immune system, the body can do the job itself without the drugs that have their toxic effects.

Along with the Hippocratic Oath that we all took, we were told *"primum, non nocere"* (first, do no harm).

4

Nutritional Research

After I had been in pediatric practice for about 20 years, I realized that medical school did not teach me everything I needed to know to be a reliable doctor. I shifted my practice to a more nutrition-oriented approach when I discovered that such conditions as bed-wetting and hyperactivity were not psychogenic, but related to diet and nutrient deficiencies. My wife and I could not tolerate the idea that these conditions in our children were the result of poor parenting skills. What a relief to know that these problems were related to nutrition and not psychogenic factors.

I found, in general, that many of these so-called "psychiatric" conditions were really genetic problems that became manifest when the diet was not appropriate. Sometimes it was the stress of bad parenting skills, poor teaching techniques, or the big dog on the way to school, plus a feeble diet that allowed a familial tendency to surface in a child.

Clinical Studies

I conducted a clinical study over ten years involving eight thousand youngsters who had been diagnosed by the teacher as hyperactive or academic failures. I discovered that 75 percent of them were blue-eyed blonds or green-eyed redheads. Boys outnumbered the girls by five to one. The hyperactivity among the few brown-eyed African–American patients was usually the result of some birth insult, like a difficult delivery. Birth injury, bilirubin toxicity, or premature birth help explain the syndrome, but most had a genetic tendency that only showed up if they were eating the wrong foods or they had a calcium or magnesium deficiency.

Most of them were very ticklish. I could hardly touch them. The stethoscope and the otoscope were like knives. I found that the response to my exam correlated well with being distractible in the classroom. Hair and blood tests showed me that the children who were distractible were also low in magnesium. Magnesium is necessary for the function of the limbic system, part of which is devoted to screening or filtering out unimportant stimuli. These children are unable to disregard unimportant stimuli. The teacher asks them to sit down and pay attention, but they are unable to do this. There are too many distractions, such as the other children in the class breathing or cars going by outside.

The other giveaway clue that the diet is faulty is that these children have mood swings, or they are a Jekyll-and-Hyde type. This syndrome is not psychiatric, but is due to fluctuating blood sugar levels. When I gave these children calcium and magnesium and had them stop the sugar or any food to which I found them sensitive, 80 percent of them were 60 to 100 percent better, and the Ritalin (a stimulant drug used to treat hyperactivity), therefore, could be discontinued.

Stephen Schoenthaler

Other confirmatory research helped me become more comfortable in saying that "hyper" kids had a nutrition problem. Stephen Schoenthaler, a professor of criminal justice in Turlock, California, has done much research to show diet is a key in maladaptive behavior in children. He conducted a now-famous investigation on New York school children. Back in 1979 he started changing the breakfasts and lunches of the 800,000 children. The first year he stopped the sugar, the next year it was the colors, then the next year it was the flavors, and then the additives. In five years he moved the average achievement test from a sad 38 up to a better than average of 53. The children who were getting the worst scores in 1979 were eating the school food; at the end of the five years, the children who were getting the best grades were eating the school food. But remember, the food had gotten better. If children eat good food, their scores improve. The brain is the busiest organ we have. It needs to be nourished or it won't work properly.

Schoenthaler went on. In a detention home for really bad boys in Oklahoma, he conducted a double-blind, crossover, placebo-controlled study on seventy-one rough, surly male adolescents.

Before the program started the administration had a list of complaints about these thugs: fights, throwing furniture, noncompliance, and escape attempts. Half of these boys got a multiple vitamin and mineral capsule; the other half got a placebo pill. Within two weeks, the kids on the vitamins became more compliant, escape attempts and fights dropped 75 percent, and surliness almost disappeared. There was a 5 percent change in the placebo group, but nothing significant. In six weeks, the placebo group got the vitamin capsule, and the incidence of antisocial behavior got better to the same 75 percent as the other group had. But the group now on the placebo began to go back to their old antisocial behavior.

This vitamin capsule cost the state about a dollar or two a week per youngster. They decided not to use it because they have Valium to control behavior, and besides, they feed these kids good food, don't they? Schoenthaler even has documentation of the vitamin and mineral status of these youngsters: hyperkeratosis, white spots on the nails, cracks at the corners of their mouths, gingival hyperemia, dilatation of the scleral capillaries.

Research has proven that diet and behavior are related. Why doesn't it happen to everyone in the same way? Vitamin and mineral deficiencies affect different people in different ways. Some people go into crime. Some get depressed. Some get sick or have headaches. Some get hyperactive, some hypoactive.

A former patient of mine just got out of federal prison after eleven years serving time for bank robbery. I took care of his pediatric needs until he was an adolescent. He was surly and uncooperative. He hated school. I tried to get him to change his diet, but he craved and stole sugar. He robbed a bank when he was twenty years old. He had not eaten breakfast that day. During the robbery he killed his uncle by mistake, and wounded a policeman. After they caught him, he could hardly remember the episode, he was so spaced-out. Remember, if you are about to rob a bank, assume it will be very stressful, and you, being a smart person, should load up with complex carbohydrates, some protein and extra C and the B-complex.

As part of the arresting procedure, the police should ask if the accused had been drinking or eating, and if so, what. Teachers know this. Most have a rule: "No child can be taught anything if he did not bring his brain to school."

Each fall I talk to the California Reading Teachers Association meeting. They always have the meeting the first week of November. Do you know why? Because it follows Halloween. They know they cannot teach the children until all the candy has been eaten up, so they get substitute teachers to baby-sit while they are away. Very little learning goes on after holidays. Easter might be just as bad. But doctors have trouble believing this, as sugar and bad nutrition do not affect every child in the same way. Also, they are not with children generally after they eat sugar as mothers and teachers are.

Archie Kalokerinos and the Aborigines

I have learned much from the reports of researchers at medical meetings but also from nutrition books. As an example, Archie Kalokerinos, an Australian medical doctor, wrote a book some years ago called *Every Second Child*. He was referring to the deaths among the aborigine children after the government doctors gave these children their DTP immunization shots. Every other child died. Archie knew it wasn't pneumonia or meningitis; it was the shots. He knew that the impoverished diet that these people were on could do nothing to support the immune system, so in the absence of the appropriate vitamins and minerals, the stress of the shots wiped them out.

On his own, he supplied each child in his district with some vitamin C. They received 100 mg. a day per month of age. A six-month-old received 600 mg.; the eight-month-old got 800 mg., and so forth. The one-year-old got 1,000 mg. a day, the two-year-old 2,000 mg. a day, and on until age five years and above, all of whom received 5,000 mg. per day. While the shots were administered, nobody died. *Nobody died.* Archie is still convinced that the DTP shots are the most likely cause of Sudden Infant Death Syndrome. (I believe that there must be at least ten reasons for SIDS, and the DTP shots administered to a baby with a truncated immune system is but one.)

So when I heard this from Archie, I began to do this in my practice. I'd give a DTP in one of the baby's muscles, and immediately would give a shot of vitamin C (50 mg) mixed with the B-complex (1 cc total fluid) in another muscle. Infants who had trouble with irritability and fever with the previous shots had no trouble with this method at all. I am convinced I shored up the immune system by this method. If the vitamin C and B-complex mixture is unavailable to parents, I have them give 1,000 mg of C, 100 mg of B_6, and 1,000 mg of calcium by mouth on the day before, the day of, and the day after the shots, no matter which ones. People who are malnourished or under some stress will have trouble with shots. So vitamins and minerals can be used prophylactically as well as therapeutically. Thank you, Archie.

As time passed I became more and more enthusiastic about megadoses of vitamin C and the B-complex as therapy. I shunned what I had been taught about the safety of antibiotics. (A rule we learned from the drug companies: Give a person with a cold some antibiotics so the secondary infection will not invade.)

Nutritional therapy was working. I billed insurance companies when I gave intravenous vitamin C, hoping they would see that this cheap, safe method was vastly superior to expensive hospital stays. What those companies were supposed to do was to alert the other doctors that Smith was on to something and why doesn't everyone do this, it would save vast sums of money? Instead, they called the Board of Medical Examiners to say that Smith was doing something unproven and unsafe, albeit cheap. The board suggested I retire. I did.

I then realized that the only way to encourage a change in our health management was to show doctors and lay people alike that there are other safe, effective, alternative methods of treatment. I discovered that the pressure from the pharmaceutical companies was so overwhelming and pervasive, that the allopathic doctor feels compelled to treat everything with drugs. Doctors tell me, "Smith, if you can get this nutrition stuff published in peer-review journals, I might believe you."

Frederick Klenner

Dr. Frederick Klenner did just that. His research began in the 1930s when he used vitamin C for almost any pathology, from viruses to germs, injuries to shock, coma to burns and snake bites. "While you are pondering the diagnosis, give vitamin C." He published his research in peer-review journals. I summarized and annotated his published papers in a book (*Clinical Guide to the Use of Vitamin C*, Tacoma, WA: Life Sciences Press, 1988).

He experimented on his own children: When one would come down with chicken pox or measles, he would give a small dose of C to help take the edge off the symptoms—maybe 200 mg two or three times a day. But his wife, Ann, upset with his experimenting, would plead, "Get them well, Fred." He would give them 1,000 mg every couple of hours, and they would be well in a day or two. Now we have the published results of his clinical studies that are decades old and published in peer-review journals. Safe and cheap. Why are the doctors not rushing to use these available methods?

Norman Cousins

I have been further encouraged by the work of the late Norman Cousins. He used to get a disease every ten years and then write a book about it. His first book was about his struggle with ankylosing spondylitis, *An Anatomy of An Illness*. This disease is very painful as it bends the victim into a pretzel-like position. He had heard about humor and vitamin C, so he talked his doctor into moving him out of the stifling hospital to a motel across the street and treat him with Groucho Marx movies and "Candid Camera" vignettes. Along with laughter therapy he was given intravenous vitamin C, at first but a paltry 10 grams, but finally moving up to 20 grams at a time. He found that if he could laugh for 20 minutes, he would have two hours of pain-free sleep. He could get the same blessed relief with the IV of vitamin C. They both had the same effect on pain. And the sedimentation rate, a test for inflammation in the body, improved by about 10 percent, a meaningful change. He fully recovered from the spondylitis, only to suffer from a devastating heart attack ten years later.

The assumption is that laughter or vitamin C encourages the brain to produce endorphins. Vitamin C is also a fighter against inflammation and helps the body make cortisol, the stress-controlling hormone from the adrenal glands.

As my practice grew I began to learn more things not taught in medical school. For example, some people feel better if they do not eat certain foods. Some children stop wetting the bed if they do not drink milk. Others control their diarrhea if they eat no wheat. Many reported that they felt better if they took certain vitamins and minerals. I discovered that hyperactive children improve with a diet change and with the addition of calcium and magnesium. I found that nutritional approaches to the control of conditions was a valid concept and that the use of prescription drugs is not always essential to health. I began to use drugs as the *last* thing on the therapeutic list. Nutritional therapy was useful, but it did not work for everyone, and when it did, its benefits were short-lived. But it did open the door to alternative methods of controlling the physiology of the body.

Naturopathic medical methods help many people, and there are no side effects, such as drugs often produce. Chiropractic adjustments are a miracle for others. Homeopathic remedies can work wonders. Acupuncture has great benefits and has been working for over four thousand years. Herbal remedies improve most who try them. These all are safe, nontoxic, and natural. I found I had *not been taught* everything in medical school I needed to know to help people feel good and remain disease free. But, as in the case of drug (or orthodox) therapy, many of these methods provided limited improvement or control. There was still something missing.

5

What Is Your Body Trying to Tell You?

READ YOUR BODY

A disease signals the body's owner that an imbalance is present. Some people get colds, some are plagued with allergies, some convulse, some break out, some are susceptible to diarrhea, while others will come down with lupus or cancer. Because no two of us are exactly alike in our disease susceptibilities, we do not have the same dietary needs. Individuals who sit at a desk all day using their brain, have different daily needs of nutrients than the steelworker. This is called "biochemical individuality," a phrase coined by Dr. Roger Williams, one of the great nutritional research pioneers.

Disease as an Opportunity

Diseases are opportunities for the victims to discover what went wrong. If people make basic, safe adjustments in their nutrient intake, they can start functioning normally, usually without the use of medications. Prescription drugs that help control symptoms and signs for the short-term are valuable for comfort; but some attention, at the same time, *must* be paid to the improper balance of nutrients that stressed the body's buffering capacity— to the point where the body's enzymes and immune systems could not function to ward off the illness.

The medical doctor with the method of drug therapy took the responsibility of disease control *away* from the patient. We accepted the concept that total health care should be in the doctors' hands, and as a consequence, we created a generation *totally* dependent upon those healing hands. It is a neat and efficient way to deal with illnesses. As time went on, however, these patients began to ask why they got sick in the first place. They had learned that drugs—albeit effective for curing acute diseases—were only masking the symptoms and signs. Present-day patients want to discover the *cause* of the problem and eliminate it.

Doctor means teacher. Some doctors have forgotten that their chief job is to educate. Without this exchange of information, people will not assume the responsibility for their own health. This book is designed to give you a little basic chemistry and physiology, so that you can take a more active role in the achievement and maintenance of their own health. Knowledge should lead to insight, and then to motivation, and then to active participation, and then to a healthier body and a happier outlook. A patient's insight, knowledge, and participation should be about 80 percent of health control. Only 20 percent or less of the health care should be in the physician's hands. The worst stress of all is the stress of the loss of autonomy. We will attempt to give some of that back to you.

Can you trust yourself more than your doctor's judgment? You live right there inside your body, and you are the best judge if something is amiss. Your doctor should be able to tell you when there is something wrong, if you have enough signs to indicate that a disease is incipient or present.

Here follow a few symptoms and signs that your doctor should be able to recognize, if you haven't already, that something is awry. Our premise is that you should be able to recognize and eliminate them yourself. These are harbingers of some physiological or metabolic screw-up that might lead to something more serious. By taking care of these minor problems, conditions, or irritations, you should be able to stop a metabolic process from developing into a disgusting, life-threatening, full-blown disease that the doctor would love to diagnose.

People are sick and tired of being sick and tired. Why are we so sick so often? Why is the incidence of chronic degenerative diseases increasing? What is cancer? Why do we have to have diseases? Do we need diseases? Is it a cruel joke being played upon us by a vengeful Mother Nature? Are there too many people on our planet and disease, crime, and death are a natural consequence of overcrowding? Is it all due to stressors, pollutants, too much noise, or too many angry people?

Solving Some Symptoms and Signs with Supplements

Some simple nutritional supplements should solve the following conditions:

SCALP:

Dandruff or seborrheic dermatitis: Too much sugar. Need essential fatty acids, B-complex, especially B_6 and paraminobenzoic acid, and selenium.
Thinning hair: On estrogen? Use B_6, folate, check for low thyroid and low stomach acid.
Much head perspiration: Vitamin D deficiency.

EARS:

Excess wax: Need essential fatty acids.
Cracks behind ears: Need B_6 and zinc.
Crease across the lobe: Possible susceptibility to cardiovascular disease.
Fluid behind eardrums, or retracted eardrums: possible food allergy.

EYES:

Cloudy lens: Cataract: possibly blood sugar problem. Bioflavonoids, Vitamins B_2, A, C, and magnesium.
Floaters: Need bioflavonoids, choline, inositol, vitamin K.
Dark circles under eyes: Food sensitivities (milk).
Dilated pupils in infants: Milk allergy.

NOSE:

Polyps: Allergy, salicylate sensitivity.
Bleeding: Food sensitivity. May need vitamin A, C, beta-carotene, bioflavonoids.

FACE:

Dilated capillaries: Alcohol ingestion, low stomach acid.
Acne: Too much sugar. Use zinc, essential fatty acids; if you are over 25 years old usually food sensitivity or low B_6.
Yellow cast to skin: Pernicious anemia, carotenemia.

(continued on page 40)

(continued from page 39)
TONGUE:

Geography tongue: Low B-complex; food allergies.
Cheilosis: Need B_2 (riboflavin), or look for food sensitivity.
Pale color: Anemia.
Canker sores: Food allergies, chocolate, walnuts, stress, and menses.
Edges scalloped: Food allergies, tension.
Drooling: Teething in child, allergy, *Candida*.

NECK:

Swollen glands behind ear: If on back of neck usually means food sensitivities.
Swollen glands under the corner of the jaw: Usually due to tonsillar infection; also food sensitivities.
Many skin tags: Check for blood sugar problems.

SHOULDER:

Sore tender spot (bursitis): B_{12} shots may help.

SKIN OF UPPER ARMS AND THIGHS:

Nutmeg grater, chicken skin: Usually vitamin A or zinc deficiency, but may be essential fatty acid deficiency, or low pancreatic enzymes.

NAILS:

Brittle, chipping, soft, splitting: Low stomach acid, low iron, and low calcium and magnesium; possible low thyroid.
White spots: Zinc deficiency.
Transverse ridges: In women: a nutrient deficiency during time of period.
Pallor: Anemia. If blue: low oxygen saturation.

HANDS:

Cracks at fingertips: Usually means low zinc.
Swollen distal joints (osteoarthritis): B_6, B_3 may help; test for allergies; avoid nightshade plants (potato, eggplant).

(continued on page 41)

(continued from page 40)
Tender, swollen middle joints: Rheumatoid; try B_3.
Carpal tunnel syndrom: B_6 can help.
Dupuytren's contracture of fourth finger: Vitamin E, check blood sugar.
Contact rash or itchy scaly rash on hands: Food allergies, soap, gloves; use zinc, essential fatty acids, C, A, E.
Warts: Use vitamin A, especially if frequent bronchitis and bumps on arms.

BREAST:

Nodular tender cysts: Stop caffeine, chocolate, cola; add E, iodine, B_6, essential fatty acids, magnesium.
Tender at sterno-costal junction: Use B_6.

ABDOMEN:

Smelly gas: Usually low stomach acid, low pancreatic enzymes, lactose intolerance, or food sensitivity.

FEET AND LEGS:

Knee swollen, grating when flexed: Try niacinamide.
Osgood-Schlatter in thirteen-year-old: Try selenium and vitamin E.
Skin dry, flaky: Use essential fatty acids.
Pain on moderate pressure over shin: need calcium, niacinamide.
Swollen ankles, protein in urine, and elevated blood pressure in pregnancy: Use B_6, magnesium, high-quality protein diet.
Varicose veins: Use fiber, vitamin E, magnesium, bioflavonoids.

These are nutritional faults that all doctors should be able to recognize before these insignificant nuisances coalesce into something serious, which could be recognized as a definite, diagnosable disease. That is when the allopathic doctor would make an entry in the chart and get out the prescription pad. It would be nice if he/she could notice these insignificant beginnings. We think if the doctor and the patient work together, and with the list of complaints, a good history, and the results of the blood test, some *real* prevention could be accomplished.

Paleolithic Diets

Anthropologists ("Paleolithic Nutrition," *New England Journal of Medicine*, January 31, 1985) have discovered that primitive people ate the foods that were available: lean meat (less than four percent fat), roots, vegetables (usually raw), grubs, eggs, fruit in season, nuts, some honey they stole from the bees, but grains were unheard of and dairy cows did not exist when humans were evolving. Two to twenty million years ago our ancestors were hunters and gatherers. The diet—when they could catch it—was good (undercooked on inside, and burned on outside), safe (except for toadstools), and healthful (those relatives of ours lived a whopping twenty to thirty years). Harvestable grains became available only twelve-thousand years ago; tooth decay and alcoholism soon followed. We know they had diseases; their bones tell us that. But were they happy and free of anxiety? No TV and no comic books. Imagine.

Weston Price

Present-day hunters and gatherers (e.g., Tasada in the Philippines) are doing reasonably well. Dr. Weston Price found isolated people and reported on them in the middle 1930s ("Nutrition and Physical Degeneration," Weston Price, Price Pottenger Foundation, La Mesa, CA). As a dentist he was primarily interested in the tooth decay rate of people living on unadulterated and unprocessed foods. He noted little tooth decay, but also found healthy, well-built bodies able to resist hypertension, appendicitis, diverticulitis, cancer, arthritis, depression, obesity, ulcers, and other "modern" diseases.

Our intestines and physiology have remained the *same* over those millions of intervening years, but impoverished diets, pollutants, contaminants, and chronic stressors have hurt us. We cannot go back to those times of running naked through field and forest trying to catch a rabbit for dinner. We have to make do with what comes from the store and the backyard garden. In addition we have become accustomed—or addicted—to our sedentary lifestyle, our sugary, greasy diet, and our reliance on the pharmaceutical industry.

As our ancestors evolved and migrated successfully into different climates and environments, dietary habits and lifestyles changed as they lived in those specific places. Your roots, your body type, and the diet you have been eating all your life will determine your needs at the present time. Being a Scot, I find oatmeal is good for me, but I won't kill for haggis. My Nordic wife will always have room for salmon.

Our ancestors did not live long enough to get some of the degenerative diseases that are so common now. However, when they *did* live beyond seventy or eighty years, they did not seem to suffer from these modern diseases. Just one hundred years ago cancer, heart attacks, arthritis, strokes, appendicitis, hiatal hernia, varicosities, diverticulitis, and osteoporosis were relatively uncommon, rarely reported, and some even unheard of. We have controlled typhoid, cholera, tuberculosis, and many parasitic diseases with better public and private health. Immunization shots have controlled diphtheria and tetanus. Oral polio drops have cut the incidence of poliomyelitis to almost zero. The statistics are mixed for whooping cough, measles, rubella, and mumps; the shots may not be doing their job.

Can we put the blame for the increased incidence of all these unwanted degenerative diseases on modern food, pollution, or the government? We have to blame genetics for the appearance of some of these conditions, but that may be just an easy excuse. I am much like my father who died of high blood pressure and a stroke when he was sixty years old, but since I know my genetic susceptibilities, I avoid salt, I exercise daily, have a different wife than my father, and I avoid stress. I have already outlived him by thirteen years, and my blood pressure is close to normal.

Some of us are genetically predisposed to high blood pressure, some of us will get diabetes, some will become obese, some develop ulcers, and some will slip into depression. Genetics determines your disease label, but your diet and lifestyle allow the condition to appear. If you look like Aunt Edith and she has arthritis, watch what she eats and how she lives, and avoid those things, or you may end up with the same family curse.

"My mother had terrible migraines," you tell your doctor. The doctor verifies the diagnosis.

"You do also." And that is about as far as he will go with you as he writes out a prescription for the latest pain killer.

Medical care has got to get better than that.

6

The Pitfalls of Nutritional Guesswork

Optimal health is not just being free of symptoms and diseases, but having a *zest for life*. If you are perfectly normal and healthy, then you are *cheerful* (without being a pest about it), *energetic* (without being hyperactive), *optimistic* (without being a Polly-anna fool).

The Perfect Person

If you are almost perfect, you do well with just seven hours of sleep, awakening refreshed. You can eat three to five well-balanced meals a day and maintain a weight consistent with your genetic inheritance. You have a fairly constant energy level from the time you arise until the time you retire. You have no great cravings for particular foods; no rushing out at 1 A.M. for choco-late, or requiring coffee on awakening before you are able to talk. You have a job with which you are comfortable; the pay could be better, but you are reasonably satisfied and look forward to work-ing most of the time. You are able to handle stressors without getting a rise in blood pressure, a headache, a canker sore, or other somatic symptoms. If you do get a symptom it lasts only a few hours or a day or so. You may have tried cigarettes, drugs, and alcohol, but they do not excite you enough that you need to continue their use. You can drink alcohol, but it has never been excessive. You have friends with whom you can laugh and joke freely. You have a sexual partner whom you trust and for whom you would do almost anything.

Because you were a cheerful and healthy baby, your parents, who even wanted you, were able to give you a good self-image because you were cooperative, slept through the night, and you smiled when they sang to you. You fit into the household rhythm. You didn't mind the vacuum cleaner vibrations, the buckling into the car-seat straps, the too-early feeding of solids, and your uncle's bad breath who often got too close with his "gootchie-goos."

There is no doubt that we are stuck with our genetic weaknesses. Genes are responsible for enzymes and enzymes are responsible for all the body's functions. Even if we are poorly endowed genetically, we can optimize the function of the enzymes we have. "The greater the concentration, the greater the rate of the reaction" is a chemical law, and means that up to a certain point, if the right vitamins and minerals are supplied in adequate amounts, the enzymes can function optimally. If an enzyme function requires magnesium, for instance, to do its job, the optimal amount of magnesium will make it easy for the enzyme to operate. A less than adequate amount will not allow the enzyme to work up to its full potential. Excess magnesium intake will *not* make the enzyme work any better if the magnesium is not in a soluble form.

Chemical Imbalances

The more we investigate the origin of symptoms, signs, and diseases, the more we find that nutrition—and specifically, the chemical imbalances in the blood and tissues—is at the bottom of what ails us. The triggering event that precipitates an actual disease may be an emotional upset or a physical injury. Something has stressed our body chemistry beyond its ability to compensate; our ability to buffer the changes accompanying stressors has been compromised by our lifestyle, which includes our diet. We are all at risk—some more, some less.

When the teacher complained that our "normal" children were out of sync with the rest of her class, we changed their diets. The trigger that led to the restless behavior seemed to be sugar ingestion, a noisy classroom, or a tough test in school. When I began to use a nutritional approach for the control of symptoms in my patients, I discovered the following:

1) If the mother described the child as a Jekyll-and-Hyde with mood swings, it was a giveaway that the child was eating sugar or something to which he was sensitive (milk, wheat, eggs, corn, soy, nuts, anything). Many children eat sugar or foods to which they are sensitive and do not become hyperactive or noncompliant. Apparently it takes the genetic tendency *plus* the inappropriate diet to make the symptom manifest. Often doctors interpret this behavioral change as a psychiatric problem. It is physiological.

2) If the child was ticklish, and the teacher said he was distractible, the child was usually deficient in magnesium and often calcium as well. It was a guess. Adding supplements to the diet helped many of them to settle down, but it did not work on all of them.

Many of these restless, goosey children loved milk and often drank two or three quarts daily. They might even steal it, they craved it so. It was surprising then that the amounts of calcium and magnesium in their hair tests were at the low end of normal. Where was it going? When they took calcium and magnesium supplements, the dairy-craving stopped. These children were "looking" for calcium, and somehow their bodies knew it was in the milk. However, the children were sensitive to dairy products (history of ear infections, colic, phlegm, asthma, and most had dark circles under their eyes). The cells lining the intestines were injured by the allergic reaction and were unable to break down the milk to retrieve the calcium. The more milk they drank, the more the intestines rejected it. A catch-22. But their bodies were trying to tell them that they needed calcium. (Anemic children often eat dirt to get iron. The eating of nonfoods is called pica. Chocolate cravers are searching for magnesium.)

Nutritionists know that if a person craves a specific food, he is probably sensitive to it. Food sensitivities usually make the blood sugar rise and fall rapidly. When the level falls, the victim will search for the food that makes him feel good. It is very much the same as an alcoholic who *has* to drink so he will not feel so awful. The sensitive person has to get the nutrient from some source that the body will not reject. Children who are denied dairy foods often will love to eat broccoli.

I thought that if I could improve the function of those lining cells, maybe the allergy would disappear and absorption improve. Since all the B-complex vitamins are necessary for digestion and intestinal enzyme function, why not try the B-complex? Oral ingestion of these vitamins was insufficient to ignite the enzyme fires; the supplements passed right on out in the stools. However, the *intramuscularly injected* vitamins transported via the circulation to the intestines revived and activated the "exhausted" digestive enzymes. Like jump-starting the car.

My Standard Shot

My standard method was to give a one milliliter injection of the B-complex containing 50 mg of each of the Bs, plus about 100 mg of C, intramuscularly, two or three times a week for about three weeks. Many of the children refused to return after that first shot. (They sting.) It worked on about 60 percent of the injectees. They told me that they had less gas, more energy, better dreams, fewer infections, and increased cheerfulness. Some had normal bowel movements for the first time in years. I had not suggested any of these improvements; when I stuck them I said, "See what happens." I was hoping to rule out the placebo effect.

But a number of patients, although initially benefited, soon realized that their symptoms were returning, or new ones developed. It was discouraging. I had no guidelines. I did not know how much, how often, and which ones of the various supplements were needed for any particular patient or problem. I also realized that I did not know when to quit the vitamin shots. Was the patient the best judge?

Although I was stumped as to how to proceed further, this avenue of treatment at least told me that injected vitamins and minerals was a valid approach to treating people as an alternative to the use of toxic drugs. It became my first line of therapy. If it worked, albeit temporarily, it suggested that nutrition and its coworker, absorption, were the keys to the patient's problem.

It was a natural transition. Without too much anxiety I was able to change my thinking from the "make-a-diagnosis-prescribe-a-drug" method to the concept that it was possible to prevent a problem using nutrition. The big and scary step was the next logical move: actually treating a disease with meganutrition after the disease had been established and diagnosed. I had read enough of the works of Adelle Davis, Roger Williams, Earl Mindell, Richard Passwater, Abram Hoffer, Linus Pauling, and Frederich Klenner to know what body clues indicated what deficiencies of the various vitamins and minerals. I began to use meganutrition orally, intramuscularly, and intravenously. And it worked, but again, not on everyone.

Vitamin A Deficiency

As a general rule, if a person is low in vitamin A, for instance, he is more likely to have rough, dry skin, acne, warts, dermatitis, dull hair, dandruff, brittle nails, night blindness, infections, and fatigue. So if I had a patient with a few of these symptoms and signs, it meant that the diet had been low in vitamin A for some time. I assumed he was A-deficient. (A blood test could confirm this.) After six weeks of 50,000 units of vitamin A daily, these symptoms and signs disappeared. Then I would advise him to take the 50,000 units but once a week, eat some carrots, and other A-bearing foods. I guessed at the dose, the length of time that he should take it, and how much he needed for the rest of his life. To be safe I also suggested the use of beta-carotene, the A precursor, if I thought his liver could convert it to the A form. I was guessing, but at least I knew in which direction to guess.

Then there were those people who had some of those symptoms, but were eating a diet full of A. What was going on? Roger Williams, author and researcher, coined the phrase, "individual biochemistry." We are all different and have different needs. It helped to explain my confusion, but did not help me find answers for the patients. For a time I used hair analyses to determine the nutritional needs of children and adults. It was good for determining the body load of heavy metals like lead, cadmium, mercury, arsenic, and aluminum. It was interesting to correlate the low levels of calcium and magnesium in the hair with symptoms of deficiencies of those elements; all hyperactive children whose hair I tested were low in calcium and magnesium. But I did not see any connection between the amount of sodium in the hair with blood pressure, for instance. Hair analyses were not consistent or reliable enough for my needs.

Food Sensitivities

I went to allergy conferences and found out that food sensitivities can *not* do everything, but they *can* do anything. Food reactions can cause migraine, ear infections, arthritis, bedwetting, weight gain, and lead to a poor immune system. Allergists tell me that 80 percent of people with food sensitivities frequently have low blood sugar attacks after they eat the foods to which they are sensitive. So I had people try a water fast: drink only water for four days. No sensitizing food meant no violent fluctuations of the blood sugar. Those that could maintain themselves through that big diet stressor felt better, albeit weakened. This did not work on everyone. Food-allergy skin tests or the cytotoxic tests are not as reliable or scientific as we have been lead to believe. However, a newer method of testing is showing promising results in continuing research. Electro-acupuncture testing according to Voll (EAV) may be the test of the future as it offers a reliable, non-invasive method of determining food sensitivities. It involves connecting the patient with a wire from an acupuncture point on his finger to a machine where extracts of the foods being tested are inserted into the circuit. Reactions are shown on a dial.

Intravenous Vitamins

I then tried intravenous vitamins hoping to overwhelm the allergy or the infection with a sudden blast of what I thought were the needed nutrients. It was dramatic for many. I could almost guarantee that I could make someone with viral pneumonia 80 percent better in six hours. I pushed people into health who had been suffering from allergies, mononucleosis, hepatitis, most viral diseases, and even many bacterial ones.

I experimented with the amounts of vitamin C à la Dr. Robert Cathcart: the sicker the patient, the bigger the dose of C. I used as much as 100 to 200 *grams* of C, diluted with water and mixed with calcium, magnesium, and the B vitamins. These large doses, suitably diluted, dripped into the patient's vein during a four-hour period. It was very satisfying to see the patient get well as I was letting the *safe* vitamin mixture run in.

But some of the patients reported that they did not feel well as the vitamins dripped in; some were irritable, or sad, or anxious. Something was still not right even though they gained temporary relief from the allergy or the infection. I did not know how to individualize the mixtures. How much of each ingredient? If the mixture was helpful, how often should it be repeated? What would be the long-term effects? I was unsure when to call a halt, or when to suggest a return visit. "You're well. Come back as needed." Many of them did not come back. Had they found someone who truly helped them, or were my megadoses so good, they did not need to return—ever?

Magnesium Dependency

For example, a fifty-year-old woman and her thirty-year-old daughter came to see me just before the Christmas holidays. Their main, common complaint was that they hated Christmas shopping because of the lights, the crowds, and the noise. "If Bing Crosby sings 'White Christmas' one more time, I'm going to pull the speaker off the wall!"

"Anything else bothering you?" The questioning revealed they were both very ticklish, sensitive, and hypervigilant. They had trouble relaxing and falling off to sleep. They both had muscle cramps in their feet and calves. I had heard these symptoms from many of my hyperactive patients over the years, and I knew that they usually meant a magnesium deficiency. So I asked the giveaway question: "Do you like chocolate?"

They came over the desk at me like an ocean wave. "Where is it?" they demanded.

"Back off, ladies. You are low in magnesium. Everything you have told me gives the deficiency away. Let me give you some intravenous magnesium, and a few other nutrients, like calcium, vitamin C, and most of the B-complex ones," I said, sucking the goodies into the syringe.

It was over in a few minutes. They noticed only the warmth of their flushed skin that the magnesium produces. When I called them in a few days, they were both ecstatic about their improvement. "We can go shopping again. It's like my space bubble has moved farther out from me; the crowds, the noise, and Bing are no longer right in my ears. We fall off to sleep without tossing and turning. The little cramps are gone. We don't have to go out at 2 A.M. to find a store to get some chocolate. But, look. We eat well. We get the four food groups. We eat our greens and some almonds—the magnesium foods. What is going on with our stupid bodies?"

Biochemical Individuality

I covered that query using Williams's concept of individual biochemistry to explain that because of their unique, genetic makeup, they needed more than the Recommended Daily Allowances (RDA). Since both mother and daughter have the same symptoms, the need is genetic. They both share some chemical imbalance in their systems that makes the magnesium unavailable to the magnesium-dependent enzymes. The lesson I was learning from patients was that many people have sicknesses because they have a nutritional dependency—not a deficiency.

So we are back to genetics. Our genes determine the chromosomes, and the latter are responsible for the presence and the efficiency of the body's enzyme systems. If the enzymes do not function, one will develop a diagnosable disease, usually one that is lurking in the family background. If we could discover the weak enzyme then we could be more specific in the application of the appropriate vitamin or mineral to make that enzyme function more efficiently. One chemical law applies here: The greater the concentration, the greater the rate of the reaction. Big doses might empower the enzymes.

Thiamin Not Good for Joannie

I treated Joannie when she was twenty years old for depression. Neither of us could understand why she was depressed. (A psychiatrist asked her why she wanted to be depressed.) "Let's try some nutrition," I said gleefully. I gave her a series of the B-complex vitamin shots to see if I could activate the enzyme system that produces the brain neurotransmitters responsible for cheerfulness. The shots worked for a few days, and then she became even more depressed. Undaunted, and scarcely loath, I tried the shots singly. First B_1, then in a few days B_2, and B_3, B_6, B_{12}, and folic were all tried separately. She was much worse after the B_1 shot ("That was the pits. Don't do that again."). She felt cheerful and energetic after the B_6, B_{12}, and the folic acid. She took a shot of just those three every few weeks for a while and then took them orally, but never took any more B_1. She feels fine on those three, but is a morose mess if she gets B_1. She must be recycling what B_1 she has through her own unique biochemical system, or she has some intestinal bacteria that are making it for her. (See the sequel to this in Chapter 7, pages 62–63.)

I was practicing educated guesswork. One cannot ignore the placebo effect here also. That is always a possibility. There is always some impact on the healing mechanism when a patient and a doctor get together. However, I knew that vitamin therapy could not be all suggestion, because I treated a score of infants and toddlers suffering from chronic nonspecific diarrhea and was able to cure 90 percent of them. These children had three to eight watery, smelly stools a day for months despite multiple diet changes. I used the B-complex shots on these children to get the digestive enzymes to restart their function. The vitamins by mouth could not work, as they passed right on out the other end before they could be absorbed by the damaged intestinal lining cells. The transit time from mouth to anus was just too rapid to allow for any significant absorption and subsequent benefit. The shots stopped the diarrhea almost overnight. (I continued them every other day for about seven to ten days.) I produced a physiological effect; it was not a psychological response. (The shots are painful despite using a local anesthetic. I cannot believe that these little babies hated the shots so much that they stopped their diarrhea just to spite me.)

Applied Kinesiology

I then became an eager student of applied kinesiology to see if that would make me more accurate in assessing nutrient needs.

The basic idea behind AK is that we all have an electrical field of force around us, much like the earth with its north and south poles, and the magnetic field. Because every cell in our body carries an electrical charge, the sum of all those little batteries creates an electromagnetic force around our whole body. If something gets near us that is a negative force, the electrical fields will indicate a change. The kinesiologist can test the muscle to find these changes.

He might place vials of different foods, toxins, drugs, vitamins, minerals, or amino acids near or on the client, and the muscle being tested will become weak or strong depending upon whether the substance is damaging or beneficial to the client. It sounds strange, but the results can be validated because they are reproducible. Kinesiologists have been able to find by testing and "asking" the body about its responses, what a particular person needs.

Try this: Have a friend hold her arm straight out from the shoulder, and then you try to push it down against her resistance while she is holding it up. You will notice a certain strength. Now have her hold a sugar bowl in her other hand and do the same pushing down on the outstretched arm. There is usually a marked difference in the ability to hold an arm out straight when sugar is nearby. Most people find that sugar, a negative food, weakens them.

Educated Guesswork: Vitamin A and B₆

Over the last fifteen years I have developed a program of *reading the body*. It is based on the assumption that the body is trying to tell the owner that there is something wrong. We simply have to be more astute at reading its signals. I made a list of the various symptoms and signs that indicate a deficiency, and although many deficiencies produce the same symptoms, it was helpful in narrowing down the problem to a few possibilities.

I have found that I need vitamin A. As a child I had warts all over my hands after the A-destroying hard measles complicated by a mastoiditis. Now if I get a cold or the flu and it settles in my chest, I take a shot of A (50,000 units) and 500,000 units orally for a few days; the infection clears up in three days instead of twenty.

The C works if the infection is from the neck up and A works if the infection is in my chest below my Adam's apple. I have always loved the A-bearing foods, like carrot, squash, and sweet potato. (I steal parsley from other diners' plates.) Ten years ago I tried 100,000 units daily by mouth for a month or so, to see if I would get the symptoms suggesting a toxic dose: the crossed eyes, the swollen liver, the headache, and the dry skin. I did lose the rough skin on the back of my upper arms, and my wife told me, "You smell better." I was rancid until I took the amount of A that I needed. I only take those big doses when I am sick enough to need them. After the most recent bout of the flu and the use of the megadoses, a plantar wart on the bottom of my foot fell off.

Here is another one solved by the educated-guess method: I saw a boy, age seven years, whose main problem was that he could not remember the sound of the letters, and, as a consequence, he could not learn to read. He seemed bright enough, but because of this difficulty, he felt he was stupid. He was developing a bad self-image and was beginning to hate school. Poor memory or poor recall is usually associated with a lack of pyridoxine (B_6). I asked him about his dreams. He shrugged his shoulders and looked puzzled. His mother answered for him, "I don't think he dreams." (Everyone does.) B_6 is necessary for the function of a brain enzyme that converts short-term memory into long-term memory during sleep.

Then I asked whether he had cradle cap as a baby. "Yes," she remembered, "but we called it 'crib-crust.'" Same thing. B_6 deficiency is associated with an oily, scaly type of eczema, called seborrhea. Aha, the plot thickens. Morning nausea? She admitted she was curled around the toilet bowl for three hours most every morning in the first three months of her pregnancy with him. "The doctor said it was the symbolic rejection of an unwanted child." Rubbish. B_6 is necessary for the optimal function of a liver enzyme that converts the active female hormones, estrone and estradiol, into a functionless breakdown product, estriol. Too much estrone, if it is not balanced by progesterone, will cause pregnancy-nausea.

I had them both take 100 mg of B_6 every day for a month. The mother reported back in just a couple of weeks that the boy was learning to read, and she seemed to have more energy, and they both were now having dreams, stupid though they were, but she could at least remember them. "How long do we take this B_6?" She had a right to know.

"Daaa," I answered. "How about quitting now and start again if dream recall is lost?" I was guessing. It was fun, but I was not the scientific doctor I thought I was when I graduated from medical school.

Then as if on cue, I received a telephone call from John Kitkoski.

7

Chemistry, the Key to a Healthy Life

BETTER LIVING THROUGH CHEMISTRY

So here I was, trapped between therapeutic principles—the standard, allopathic prescription-writing method, and the shaky, guesswork approach of natural, nontoxic healing based largely on anecdotal evidence. It was almost prophetic that John Kitkoski called to see if I was interested in the Life Balances Health Program.

He made chemical sense. I was hooked when he told me that the blood tests correlate almost exactly with client's senses of smell and taste. If he tends to crave dairy products, and calcium is low in the blood test, the person involved will like the smell of the calcium tablets.

Most of these concepts seemed valid since he had based them on solid chemical laws. I couldn't help but ask, "You mean, if I crave chocolate, I need it because I have a chocolate deficiency? I have a little trouble accepting that as science."

He countered with, "Chocolate has magnesium in it. If you love chocolate, you probably need magnesium." A blood-magnesium level does not always reflect magnesium needs or the amount of tissue magnesium. But the GGT (Gamma Glutamyl Transpeptidase, see Chapter 10, page 104) is produced only in the presence of magnesium. In general, the more the magnesium in the system, the higher the GGT—if liver and biliary pathology have been ruled out. I have been delighted to see the connection between chocolate craving and magnesium deficiency. If the

GGT test is low (below 25) in the blood test of a person, she usually craves chocolate, and will love the smell of the magnesium tablets. She needs magnesium, and not chocolate. Stressors to the body diminish the tissue magnesium. Many women will "kill" to get some chocolate before their periods. They are looking for the magnesium, just as calcium-deficient people may crave dairy products. This is one of the validations between the blood tests, a person's cravings, and the scores on the smelling part of the Life Balances program.

The Alkaline Dog

One day this researcher, John Kitkoski, visited my partner and noticed his well-fed but aging Airedale. "I see Shane is in alkalosis," he said without hesitation.

"Huh?"

"Do you see how shallowly and infrequently he is breathing?"

"I guess so."

"He is conserving his CO_2 by not breathing deeply. Let's try an experiment." He put three feeding dishes on the floor. He put water in one (neutral). He placed a teaspoon of vinegar in about eight ounces of water in the second one (acidic), and the third contained milk (alkaline). The dog smelled each one, and—you guessed it—he only drank the vinegar-spiked water. The dog looked up and gave us a wry smile as if to imply, "It's about time."

Doctors know, but Kitkoski had to remind me, that if someone breathes deeply and rapidly, he is trying to get rid of the CO_2 (acidic) so he will become more neutral. He may have become acidic from running and burning calories, which make CO_2 and lactic acid, or he swallowed a large dose of aspirin (acidic), and the body is trying to compensate by exhaling the CO_2. (A person in acidosis cannot hold his breath longer than a minute. An alkaline person can hold his breath longer than a minute.)

The Alkaline Human

This vinegar experiment reminded me of my wife who has been putting an ounce of vinegar on my salads for forty-four years. "It's good for you," she claims as she turns to get a pickle and I wring out the lettuce leaves.

I was getting the "AHA!" feeling; things were coming together. It made sense. Julie had trouble nursing our children because her tendency to alkalosis prevented the milk from being soluble enough to pass through her milk ducts. We both tend to have allergies and muscle cramps. I thought people took calcium and magnesium to control muscle spasms, but those chemicals tend to make one more alkaline.

We gained insight into this acid/base balance one night when we found some ice cream in our freezer. (Some burglar must have left it.) We couldn't throw it out, so we had a small helping. We then brushed our teeth, flossed, took some calcium and magnesium, went to bed, and fell asleep. We both awakened at about 2 A.M. by severe, sharp, cramping pains in the muscles of our calves and feet. We leapt around the room to work out the spasms.

"How come? We took our calcium and magnesium!" It dawned on me. The ice cream must have set up a barrier to prevent the minerals from getting into our circulation. We are both sensitive to dairy products; the ice cream with its sugar must have hurt the absorptive areas of the intestinal lining.

I checked with our researcher. "You're not exactly right. The ice cream tends to make tissues somewhat alkaline, so the calcium and magnesium would be relatively insoluble. You both need to be acidified." He suggested ammonium chloride, the salt of a weak base (alkali) and a strong acid; it is called an acidifier. Under the influence of this safe, cheap chemical, we suffer no more cramps. Even allergies are less prominent.

Clearly this researcher was on to something. He has found that the majority of us, black, white, yellow, red, brown, so-called normal people in North America are alkaline to some degree. Alkalinity tends to encourage the onset of diseases characterized by muscle tension: high blood pressure, asthma, migraine, backaches, and spastic colon.

The pH of Saliva and Urine

I knew about the use of pH paper to check the acidity of the saliva and urine so that people can regulate their acid/base balance at home. (It makes some sense but is not as accurate as the Life Balances program that depends upon the senses of smell and taste.) The lower the number on the pH scale, the more acid; the higher the number, the more alkaline. Water is neutral at seven; venous blood needs to be slightly alkaline at a pH of 7.4. The normal pH of urine and saliva are about 6.5, slightly acid. If the pH drops below that, the person is to eat mainly cooked vegetables, as they tend to increase the alkalinity. If the pH rises above the 6.5 value, the person is to eat raw fruits and vegetables, as they are more acidic. With this method the person is to find the right balance of acid-forming and alkalinizing foods to get the pH of those fluids to stay at that 6.5 level. The proper balance in the pH should allow for health as the enzymes work best at the proper pH.

You can buy this pH paper at the pharmacy and test your saliva and urine. The trouble with this method is that fruits and vegetables, cooked or raw, no matter what their initial pH value, will be metabolized eventually to vinegar in the body. Sometimes your system is alkaline but your secretions are acidic—and vice versa. The method is flawed, although it can give some temporary relief.

My researcher friend also told me about his twenty-five years of animal research and the vast database he accumulated showing the correlation of the blood tests with the disease signs. The chemical laws are equally applicable to plants and animals. His research indicated that for his program he needed twenty or so main nutrients that humans do not get consistently in their daily food intake. He found the purest possible nutrients, so that no binders or fillers would interfere with the pure, individual odor of each vitamin or mineral.

Smell Your Way to Health

The client smells the contents of each bottle in a special sequence. The odor is scored on a scale of 1 to 10.

- 1 is sweet; it really smells good
- 2 is good and mildly sweet
- 3 is no smell, as if the bottle is empty
- 4 is a slight odor, not particularly good or bad
- 5 is a borderline odor, but is not bad

- 6 is slightly offensive
- 7 is a definite turnoff; most wrinkle their noses at this
- 8 is pretty bad
- 9 is very offensive
- 10 is a real stink; it is called pukey. Nauseating

As the bottles are being smelled, the scoring numbers are recorded on a sheet. If the score is a 5 or less, it means the client needs that one that day, so he swallows one tablet. If a 1, the subject is really deficient in that nutrient, so he takes it, but it also means he is to go through the bottles twice more that day. If the score is a 2, the program is to be resmelled once more that day. That low a score indicates a strong need. **Example:** I notice that the bottle of vitamin D has a repulsive smell to me in the summer, but after about November, it gets to be a no-smell (3) or a sweet smell (2). I don't need vitamin D in the summer, but I do need it in the winter.

If any one of the bottles has a bad or disgusting odor (sometimes associated with a "Yuk!" exclamation), it means that the person got enough from his food that day, or his body has it naturally. The smeller is not to take it—at least that day. **Example:** if I have eaten some milk, cheese, or ice cream on Monday, Tuesday the bottle with the calcium smells like used kitty litter, a definite 9. By Thursday without dairy products, the calcium score will move down to a 3 or 4, and I will need it again. It is interesting that many people who crave milk and drink more than a quart a day still find the calcium smells good. It suggests that they are not able to absorb the calcium from the milk; their sensitivity to milk impairs the absorption of the calcium.

One of the bottles in the program contains pills of the acidifier, ammonium chloride, the salt of a weak base and a strong acid. (Not all drug stores have this, but the Life Balances office will supply a bottle for your use. It comes as a 7½ grain tablet.) If a person is alkaline, he usually loves the smell of it. Julie says it smells like vanilla, so I then give her two or three of them. In about thirty minutes when she smells it again, it has a bad, sickening smell to her. She has had enough for the time being. Sometimes I awaken her when I go to bed at midnight, and have her smell the ammonium chloride. She usually says, "I don't smell anything." So I give her two of them. If I do not, she is likely to awaken at 3 A.M. with a terrible muscle cramp in her calf. She assumes that if I were a better husband, she would not need these vitamins and minerals. The acidifier makes the calcium soluble enough to allow muscles to relax. She likes me if her chemistry is good, and loves me if her pH is perfectly balanced.

This subjective method of determining what one needs by using the sense of smell means that one never over- or underdoses. The nose is a surveillance mechanism to alert the body that something good or bad is about to enter. "Take appropriate action. Accept or reject! You have five seconds to decide."

Here is another "AHA!" Health-store managers tell me that many people will buy an all-inclusive vitamin and mineral formula that contains forty-plus nutrients. After about a month has gone by, however, the customer comes back with his partially used bottle. He says, testily, "Hey, this was working for a couple of weeks, and now they don't seem to be doing any good, and the pills smell bad. I think the vitamins have gone sour. I want my money back." The manager takes a whiff. "It smells the same as when you bought it. Here's a fresh, unopened bottle from the same company. I'll open it." Manager smells contents. "It smells just like your bottle. It is the same stuff, and it has not spoiled." The point here is that the *person*—not the supplements—has changed. Some of the nutrients in the pills the customer ingested became an overdose after about two or three weeks, and the nose/body connection was trying to signal the body's owner to stop taking them. Many of the nutrients in the pills are still necessary for the customer, but the overwhelmingly disgusting smell of the overdosed ones makes it impossible to differentiate the needed from the unneeded.

It can be a boring drag to have to smell each of the nutrients every day, but it is important that only the ones needed are taken. Remember Joannie (see page 52) to whom I gave those mixed vitamin B and C shots about twelve years ago? They helped to lift her depression for a while, but then they stopped working. I was sure she had an endogenous depression as there was nothing in the history to indicate that it was stress, or family, or her boyfriend. She, however, knew that there were some good things about the shots, so she suggested to me that I give the B vitamins separately.

I gave her 100 mg of B_1, and followed that in three or four days with 100 mg of B_2, then B_3, then B_6, then B_{12} (1 mg), and finally folic acid (10 mg). B_1 had a bad effect on her, B_2 nothing, nor did

B_3, but after the B_6 shots she said, "I think you are on to something." Then the B_{12} and the folate gave her a definite lift. So we just gave her the B_6, B_{12}, and folic acid. No more depression.

Time passes. Last year she was thirty-one years old, happily married, and with her same good job, but she was slipping into her depression again. Instead of giving the shots, I had her smell each bottle, to see which were her favorites. Most of the vitamins and minerals had some odor to them, but nothing really sweet nor terribly offensive, until she came to the bottle of thiamine (B_1). "Good Lord," she exclaimed, "it smells as if I have my head in the toilet! There's something wrong with this bottle." No, Joannie, it's you. You don't need thiamine today. Apparently she has bacteria in her intestines, which manufacture thiamine, and then she absorbs what she needs. When she takes thiamine, she gets depressed.

There are many of us who are taking too much of one vitamin or mineral, and not enough of the others. With Life Balances there is no more guesswork.

If the body is perfectly balanced and all the nutrients are present in the right proportion, sicknesses, mental and physical, are easily dealt with. We all know that vitamin C does many wonderful things, but one of those things that has not been explored is that it acts as an acid, and when one takes C as the ascorbic acid, it may be acting to acidify the ingester, and hence correcting an alkaline condition. The right amount of C can help make iron more bioavailable, but too much C can wash it out of the body.

This whole book is based on the concept that since we cannot go back to the way we are meant to be in the hunting and gathering days of two million years ago, we have to make do with what we've got. You may not *want* to go back to those dear dead days; the average length of life was but twenty to thirty years. Even if we eat food that is whole and natural, we will still not get what we need because of the topsoil's depletion of so many of the nutrients. Most of us need only fifteen hundred to three thousand calories a day, depending on our exercise level; if we were working enough to use four thousand calories a day, we might get close to taking in the optimum amounts of nutrients. Even if we ate the best of the high nutrient-dense foods, we would become deficient in some of the vitamins and minerals because of stressors, allergies, and imperfect absorption. We all need supplements. But how much and which ones?

8

Your Senses Tell Your Needs

CLUES ABOUT VITAMIN

AND MINERAL DEFICIENCIES

The olfactory or smelling sense helps to indicate deficiencies or excesses. John Kitkoski spent considerable time and effort to find laboratories that manufacture the purest products available. When you open a bottle from the kit, what you smell is what is on the label. What you smell is what you get. Many people like the smell of a particular vitamin or mineral and yet they have no symptoms suggesting a deficiency. It suggests, however, that some problem is on its way.

But the Life Balances program will not work if an individual uses the traditional ''one symptom means one deficiency'' method. The LB approach to health is a hard concept for many of us to grasp. Kitkoski believes that an illness is not a particular vitamin or mineral deficiency but a complex relationship between ratios. He uses examples like the comparison of a cake and a brownie recipe.

The difference between a cake and a brownie recipe is the ratio of eggs to flour. An illness is no different from a recipe. If a cake calls for a cup of flour and you are missing one-third cup of flour, you simply add the proper amount to finish the cake. The problem with an illness is that you may or may not have more than one thing out of balance. Your chemistry is unique and your recipe is as unique as a snowflake. Nevertheless, the following examples of slight and gross deficiencies of the various vitamins and minerals should help one see the connection of the olfactory and gustatory senses to the body's needs. The neurons in the brain can sense changes of the metabolites in the plasma and will fire slower or faster or allow a greater number of neurotransmitters to be released.

Roger J. Williams, Ph.D., professor of chemistry at the University of Texas, wrote this in 1956: "Each human individual has quantitatively a distinctive pattern of nutritional needs . . . from individual to individual, specific needs may vary severalfold." He tried to teach us that nutrition is for *real* persons with all their nutritional variability. Calcium needs in different individuals can vary by a factor of four, and some vitamins by a factor of forty. The Life Balances program individualizes the vitamin and mineral needs, because of its reliance on the senses of smell and taste.

The vitamins and minerals serve as facilitators of enzyme functions. The need is dependent upon the metabolism of the individual. They are not stored to any great extent, so they need to be replaced almost daily.

Deficiency Symptoms and Signs

Vitamin A. If the contents of the vitamin A bottle smell good, or there is no smell, it suggests you need it at the time you smell it. People who need A have usually had: stress, asthma, fevers, frequent colds, bronchitis, inner ear disease, diabetes, cortisone use, smoking or exposure to pollutants, trauma, cancer, digestive disturbances, alcohol ingestion, pregnancy, liver problems. In a government study a few years ago, 40 percent of youths under the age of seventeen years had vitamin A levels below acceptable amounts.

Most people who think the A smells good have had the following: dermatitis, rough dry skin, warts, acne, ulcers (skin or duodenal), dull hair, dandruff, brittle nails, softening of bones and teeth, loss of appetite, diarrhea, heavy menstrual flow, red, scaly, dry eyelids, conjunctivitis with pus, poor night vision, sensitivity to glare.

Vitamin B_1 (Thiamine). If this vitamin smells good, or there is no smell, it means the smeller needs it at that time. A need for B_1 is usually associated with excess sugar ingestion or a poor diet, smoking, alcohol ingestion, fever, stress, trauma, and diarrhea.

If a person has a need of thiamine, B_1 usually smells good to them, and they may have any or all of these: fatigue, weakness, depression, paranoia, reduced ambition, irritability, anxiety, insomnia, confusion, memory loss, learning disability, numbness and tingling of hands and feet, clumsiness, increased sensitivity to noise and pain, anorexia, heart irregularity, abdominal pain.

Vitamin B_2 (Riboflavin) is needed if processed food is prominent in the diet, stress, trauma, pregnancy, lactation, need for high energy, fever, antibiotic use.

If a person is low in riboflavin, the contents of the B_2 bottle will have no smell or a good smell. They might have some of the following: fatigue, depression, dizziness, weight loss, photophobia, red cracked lips, burning eyelids, dermatitis, magenta-colored tongue.

Vitamin B_6 (Pyridoxine) is needed if one is on a poor diet or a fast, is pregnant, using oral contraceptives, has infections, getting radiation, or having stress.

The tablets of B_6 will smell good or have no smell if memory and dream recall is poor, there is fatigue, muscle weakness, irritability, nervousness, depression, somnolence, dizziness, numbness, pain, tingling, headaches, low blood sugar, dandruff, seborrhea, eczema, premenstrual syndrome, asthma, allergies, infertility, anemia, stiff joints, cheilosis, conjunctivitis, geography tongue, stunted growth, poor wound healing, carpal-tunnel syndrome, hyperactivity, kidney stones.

Vitamin B_{12} (Cyanocobalamin) is needed if one is a smoker, a strict vegetarian, a chronic laxative user, or has heavy bleeding.

These tablets usually have a sweet or no smell to those with pernicious anemia, neuritis, weakness, fatigue, depression (especially postpartum), irritability, memory loss, confusion, headache, dizziness, moodiness, asthma, malabsorption, numbness and tingling, soreness, beefy redness of tongue, anorexia, constipation, postural hypotension, body odor, palpitations, yellow pallor to skin, psychosis, paranoia.

Vitamin C (Ascorbic acid) is needed if one is a smoker or exposed to pollutants, stress, injuries, fevers, infections, excessive physical activity, burns, antibiotic use, drugs, addictions, cortisone, or there is anemia, cancer, arthritis.

The tablets of vitamin C smell good to those who are alkaline, or irritable, fatigued, anxious, have anorexia, indigestion, easy bruisability, loose teeth, bleeding gums, slow wound healing, hair loss, dyspnea, gallstones, allergies, anemia, susceptibility to infections.

Vitamin D (from fish oil) is needed if there is a lack of sunshine, one is on a low-fat diet, or a high phosphorus diet (meat and soft drinks), pregnancy, lactation, adolescence, a vegan diet (a strict vegetarian diet that proscribes dairy products as well as animal flesh), menopause, malabsorption.

The capsules often smell good to participants during the winter and smell bad during the summer because of the excess or lack of exposure to the sun; osteoporosis, osteomalacia, soft nails, irritability, nervousness, insomnia, muscle cramps, joint pain, large number of cavities, burning in mouth and throat, diarrhea, myopia, sweaty scalp.

Vitamin E (Tocopherol) is needed if one is exposed to tobacco smoke or pollutants, drugs, stress, vigorous exercise, chronic ingestion of cooked, unsaturated fats and processed food, chronic laxative use.

The capsules smell good to many who have anemia, diabetes, elevated cholesterol, low hormone production, low sex drive, infertility, premenstrual syndrome, menstrual difficulties, diseases of liver, kidneys, pancreas, ulcerative colitis, malabsorption, ulcers, muscle swelling or wasting, brittle or falling hair, lupus, gout, arthritis.

Biotin is needed if one is on a very poor diet, during pregnancy, lactation, or there is malabsorption or stress. The tablets usually have no smell and most people get it from most any diet. Those who need it may be fatigued, depressed, have a scaly, gray-looking dermatitis, seborrhea, eczema, cheilosis, a smooth magenta-colored tongue, insomnia, muscle pains, nausea, vomiting, infections, anemia, hypercholesterolemia.

Choline is needed if one is on a very poor diet, has malabsorption, stress.

These tablets usually smell like three-day-old dead fish to most participants, so they do not want it nor need it. If it smells good or there is no smell, people usually have one or some of these: poor memory, confusion, vagueness, high cholesterol, arrhythmias, fat intolerance, gastric ulcers, growth retardation, hypertension, liver impairment, kidney disease, eczema.

Calcium is needed if one gets little sunshine, is on a poor diet (no dairy, and no vegetables), low-fat diet, or has malabsorption.

If the tablets have no smell or smell good, one would most likely have muscle cramps, arm and leg numbness, tingling of lips, tongue, fingers, feet, carpopedal spasm, sensitivity to noise, and be prone to tooth decay. A severe deficiency: rickets, convulsions, laryngospasm.

Folic Acid is needed if oral contraceptives used, not eating leafy vegetables, has excess alcohol ingestion, parasites, bleeding, cancer, stress, malabsorption, diarrhea. Any condition resulting in the increase need for blood formation will increase the need for folic acid.

These tablets have little smell for most, but would smell good if one has megaloblastic anemia, numb, weak, unstable, restless legs (like B_{12} deficiency). Might have smooth, sore, red tongue, mouth ulcers, dizziness, apathy, forgetfulness, anorexia, graying hair, growth retardation.

Betaine Hydrochloride is a stomach acid substitute and would be good for those with cancer, old age, low serum iron, chronic use of antacids and gastric acid inhibitors. The body will not be able to absorb B_{12}, folic acid, the eight essential amino acids, and all the minerals without sufficient HCl.

Most people think these tablets really stink because they have enough stomach acid. Those who need this, and to whom these smell good usually have dyspepsia and foul-smelling gas, much belching, unable to digest protein, slowed bowel motility, food sensitivities, protein deficiency, parasites, pernicious anemia, soft nails, thin hair.

Iron is needed if one is on a diet high in phosphorus, if low in stomach acid, on antacids, a poor diet (much milk, white bread, and white rice), chronic use of tea and coffee, high amounts of cellulose in the diet, bleeding ulcers, and heavy menstrual flow, chronic and repeated infections, rapid growth, pregnancy.

These tablets will smell sweet to those who are anemic (microcytic), constipated, pale, fatigued, confused, depressed, dizzy, have cold hands and feet, headaches, anorexia, irritability, dyspnea, brittle concave nails, sore tongue, paresthesias of hands and feet, heart palpitations, low stomach acid, skin sores, fragile bones, pica (eating ice or dirt), flatulence, nausea, epigastric distress with belching.

Magnesium is needed if one is on a poor diet with no green vegetables, nuts, or seeds; or if have stress, diarrhea, diabetes, kidney disease, malabsorption, on diuretics, or are alcoholics.

This has no smell or a good smell if one has a deficiency: apathy, irritable nerves and muscles, apprehension, weakness, confusion, depression, hyperactivity, paranoia, anorexia, nausea, vomiting, sensitivity to noise, irregular heart beat, ticklishness, chocolate craving, muscle cramps and twitches in feet and legs, insomnia, hypothermia, hand tremors, body odor.

Vitamin B_3 (Niacin, niacinamide) is needed if one drinks alcohol excessively, or eats much sugar, starches, is engaged in strenuous exercise, has trauma, or pregnancy, rapid growth, antibiotic use.

This will smell good or have no smell to those who need it. Deficiency clues: fatigue, confusion, depression, irritability, loss of sense of humor, paranoia, hypoglycemia, memory loss, crying jags, anorexia, dyspepsia, diarrhea, tender gums, red, scaly dermatitis, high cholesterol, headaches, ringing in the ears, insomnia, unmanageable hair, canker sores, cheilosis, sore, red tongue, low stomach acid, halitosis, arthritis.

Paraminobenzoic Acid is needed if one is eating poorly or has malabsorption.

This often has no smell, and rarely smells bad. If one needs it one might have gray hair, vitiligo, wrinkles, eczema, arthritis, scleroderma, depression, irritability, nervousness.

Pantothenic Acid is needed if one is on a very poor diet, has much stress, has used cortisonelike drugs, or has malabsorption.

If the tablets smell good, there may be a possible deficiency and coordination would be impaired, faintness on arising, joint and muscle pain, fatigue, insomnia, weakness, allergies.

Ammonium Chloride (NH_4Cl) is the salt of a weak base and a strong acid, hence, it is an acidifier. One would need this if one is alkaline and the nitrogen elements in the blood test are low. Alkaline foods often bring this about, but aging is a factor.

If this smells good, the participant is usually alkaline, often loves vinegar, may be fatigued, has various muscle aches, asthma, spastic colon, migraine.

These are the main vitamins and minerals that are used in the program. Participants are to go through the kit daily, smelling each bottle in turn and taking those that are good smelling, have no smell, or a barely detectable one.

Included in the program are six dropper bottles of minerals: potassium, zinc, magnesium, copper, chromium, and manganese. A specific number of drops from each bottle are mixed in a glass of orange, apple, or some acidic fruit juice as the minerals are more soluble in an acidic medium. The drink is swallowed once a day, usually with breakfast. If the juice with its added minerals does not taste good—too sour, metallic, disgusting—it means that one of the minerals is not appropriate to that participant's metabolism on that particular day and it is discontinued until the inappropriate one is discovered by tasting them all individually.

A gentleman who knew he was overloaded with copper from a toxic water pipe in his home had only to taste about a teaspoonful of the juice with the drops in it to tell us that it was not right. He spat it out immediately when it hit his taste buds. He will not need copper for a long time to come.

The minerals are usually needed for people who have nutrient deficiencies.

Potassium is needed if one is on a low-fruit and vegetable diet, or diuretics, or on a high sodium diet. It will reduce the diastolic blood pressure if it is above 90 mm mercury.

If potassium drops do not change the taste of the juice, then potassium is a good idea, especially if one has muscular weakness and soreness, twitches, erratic and rapid heart beats, fatigue, insomnia, edema, electrocardiogram changes, glucose intolerance, hypercholesterolemia.

Zinc is needed if one is on a low-zinc diet (common). Starvation, anorexia, constant use of unleavened bread. If zinc is available to the body, bones grow in length.

Rarely do the zinc drops change the taste; it is needed daily. Zinc is low in these problems: anemia, depressed cell-mediated immunity, iron deficiency, poor growth, hypogonadism (delayed sexual maturation), infertility, impotency, prostate swelling, anorexia, acne, dysgeusia (distorted taste sensation), diarrhea, apathy, birth defects, slow growing and brittle nails and hair, hair loss, depression, eczema, fatigue, stretch marks, hypercholesterolemia, poor wound healing, malabsorption, memory loss, white spots on nails (see symptoms under A deficiency). A zinc shortage may allow aluminum to get into the brain. Zinc is a vital component of enzymes in the brain which repair worn-out cells. If these enzymes do not get all the zinc they need, dementia may begin.

Copper is needed for iron metabolism and hemoglobin synthesis, is involved in neurotransmitter formation, is an antiinflammatory agent.

A deficiency is seen with anemia, leucopenia (low WBC count), osteoporosis, bone spurs, depigmentation, weak nails, low body temperature, sparse, brittle or kinky (closely twisted) hair.

Chromium is needed to make insulin more efficient in carbohydrate metabolism.

A deficiency would show up as glucose intolerance, weight loss, mental confusion.

Manganese is needed for carbohydrate metabolism, growth, reproduction, energy production. If manganese is available to the body, bones grow in diameter.

A deficiency may show as weight loss, dermatitis, nausea, vomiting, changes in hair color, a low cholesterol, makes one prone to athletic injuries, strained knees, bone deformities.

Most people on the program will go through the twenty bottles of vitamins and minerals each day. They will smell each in turn, taking a tablet if the contents smell good or if there is no smell, and not taking them if the contents have a disagreeable odor. Most participants, after a few weeks, find that they not only feel better, or have fewer symptoms, but will find their scores get closer to 4s, 5s, or 6s.

One man with full-blown AIDS loved the smell of each of the twenty bottles, he was so deficient. "What is this?" he said with enthusiasm despite his fever and lethargy. "It smells so sweet— like a spring day. The clouds have parted and the sun is shining through." He needed all of them. He scored them all as 1s.

In two weeks on the program his fever and swollen glands had returned to normal, and he got by on twelve hours of sleep instead of twenty-five. As he recovered the smelling scores rose to 3s and 4s.

The body knows what it needs.

WHAT YOU CAN DO FOR YOURSELF

If you have any of the symptoms listed under the specific vitamins or minerals, you could launch—in an amateurish way—your own program. For example, you notice that you have too many infections. The list indicates that you might need vitamins A, C, biotin, and possibly iron. You then go to the health food store and buy the bottles with those items in each of four separate bottles. When you open the bottles, they should smell good or at least have no smell to you. You take the indicated amounts—usually one pill each day—and see if you feel any better in a month or six weeks. Remember, you are *guessing* about your needs, but it is an educated guess, and even borders on science.

Here is another: You have skin trouble. Any or all of the following might be involved with skin health: A, zinc, essential fatty acids, B_2, B_3, B_6, C, biotin, choline, and PABA. You next buy these items as separate entities, and not as a B-complex. Again when you open the bottles, the contents should smell good or have little or no smell. Choline stinks to most of us.

One more: You are anxious, fatigued, weak, tense, or depressed and have some insomnia. You are ticklish and have muscle cramps. You probably need B_1, B_2, B_6, biotin, calcium, magnesium, and B_3. Again the contents should smell good or have little or no smell, if you have chosen the proper ones, and the contents of the bottles are as pure as possible.

You must be aware, however, that nutrition "therapy" is not like drug therapy, which says one treatment for one disease (i.e., penicillin for strep throat). Vitamins and minerals work in concert and the ratios between the items may be more important than the amounts. You may not have success with this "guessing game" because you need the electrolyte solution to help carry the goodies into your bloodstream and then on to the enzymes, waiting in the distance cells.

But it can be fun. It is usually safe and these methods might help you. It would also be nice if health stores would make available samples of pure vitamins and minerals so customers could take a whiff and determine their needs as of that day before they make a purchase.

9

A Trace of Science for the Chemically Naive

IF YOU KNOW THAT H₂O IS WATER, YOU UNDERSTAND CHEMISTRY.

I loved chemistry in college and medical school and I got good grades. We saw some exciting connections between the lab results and the patients' diseases, which helped to establish the diagnosis, our main job as doctors. (E.g., 400 mg of blood glucose means diabetes; hemoglobin of eight grams equals anemia; pus in the urine reveals a kidney infection; lower right quadrant pain plus an elevated WBC suggests appendicitis.)

However, no one taught us the interrelatedness of these laboratory tilts to the patients' symptoms, unless the symptoms were quite obvious. Fatigue or disagreeableness were not connected consistently with any specific lab work that led us to the diagnosis. We dumped all of those into the psychoneurotic basket.

Chemistry is the Study of Matter

We struggling clinicians need medical truisms or laws. The vagaries of human metabolism defy classification. We are told we are scientists; we need a structure of the material universe (animals, plants, earth, air), which explains all that goes on in it and from that framework predict behavior after any given change. We are not satisfied to accept phenomena on faith. We want every symptom, thought, feeling, breath, and action of a patient to be based on facts: millions of molecules and ions are at work, acting in a predictable way. Chemistry is that framework: It provides a model of the working of the universe in terms of which all events can be explained. Humans are part of that universe. Chemistry is the study of the matter of which the universe is built.

Metals, drugs, gasoline, pesticides, food, the earth, and human cells all have properties determined mainly by chemical principles. Everything is ruled by chemical laws.

Chemistry is basically electricity. There are ninety-two elements that have been identified. Each atom is unique because each has a different number of protons and neutrons in the nucleus at its center, and a balancing number of electrons whizzing around that center in different orbits. We know that the smallest particles of matter, the atoms, can neither be formed nor destroyed; the numbers of atoms of any kind are the same in the reactants as in the products. Atoms become ions if they gain or lose electrons. The bonds between ions is the attraction between two electrical charges. The strong links between atoms allows them to become molecules—tightly bound atomic clusters. These links are chemical bonds; they are the most crucial step in the architecture of matter. Here is how nature makes table salt. When sodium (Na) combines with chlorine (Cl) it has to transfer an electron from its outer shell to the outer shell of the Cl.

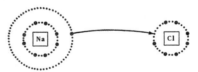

The electron fills the outer shell and the two atoms become a molecule. The closed shell is more stable and is preferred by nature. If an atom does not have a closed shell, it attempts to achieve one; atoms with incomplete shells will interact with other atoms in such a way that each partner completes its outer shell. These + and − charges must exactly balance. Sodium, a cation as Na +, and Chloride, an anion as Cl −, have shared an electron and thus the electron needs of two atoms are satisfied. These bond changes, which lead to the change in the composition of matter, are called chemical reactions.

Na plus Cl has now become table salt. When salt is dropped into water it dissociates into ions with a charge, sodium (Na +) and chloride (Cl −). The link is due solely to the electrical forces between the charged ions. The bond is the attraction between two opposite electrical charges, called ion pairs. The electro-negativity of the elements is the property that decides the facility with which an atom gains or loses electrons. If electronegativity is high, the atoms attract additional electrons and so form anions. Atoms of low electronegativity readily lose electrons and easily form cations, (positive +); their outer shells contain only one or two electrons.

Therefore, the properties of the atoms are a reflection of the activity of the electrons in the outer shells. Linus Pauling is quoted as saying as an extension of that, "The properties of living organisms are those of aggregates of molecules." Life must consist of the ordering of atoms into molecules in the cells and the further interaction of those molecules to do the work of the cells. Thousands of atoms form in a special way to become enzymes. These enzymes act as biological catalysts to aid the shift of electrons from old bonds to new ones.

Electrolytes are atoms with a charge, either a positive (+) or a negative (−) charge (see Chapter 13). All acids are electrolytes and have H+ ions when in solution. We learned in college chemistry, "pH is the negative log of the hydrogen ion concentration," which means that on a logarithmic scale of 0 to 14, with 7 (water) as neutral, the lower the number, the more acidic or the more H+ ions are available. The higher the number the more basic or alkaline is the solution, and the fewer the H+ ions and the more OH− ions. Stomach acid is about 2 to 3. Arterial blood is 6.4, and venous blood is 7.42, slightly alkaline.

Ammonium chloride (NH_4Cl) has been mentioned. This is a salt of a weak base and a strong acid. In solution it breaks down to: NH_4+ plus Cl− and $H_2O > H+$ plus Cl− plus NH_4+ and OH− and becomes an acidifier because the H+ ions are released in greater quantity than the OH− ions. (The NH_4 bonds more readily to the OH than the H bonds to the Cl.)

Oxidation is the addition of oxygen to an element or a compound, or a reaction in which hydrogen is removed from a compound. Reduction is the opposite: Hydrogen is added or oxygen is removed.

You can see that chemistry is basically about electrons, neutrons, protons, and electrostatic forces between atoms. The properties of the atoms depend upon the mass of the positive nucleus and the magnitude of that charge, and the configuration of the electrons. A million atoms lined up would just stretch across the period at the end of this sentence. Tiny as the cell is, the atoms are about ten thousand times smaller. (A look at relative sizes: if the nucleus of an atom is the size of a golf ball, the first electron in the inner shell rotating about it would be a *kilometer* away. It is mostly empty space inside those atoms.)

Every cell with its dissolved minerals provides the electrical energy—like a tiny battery—that is required to do the work of the body. One-third of the energy of the body is required just to pump sodium out and potassium into the cells to make the electrical gradient. (This pump works better if potassium is supplied in greater amounts than sodium.) The electrocardiogram and the electroencephalogram are used to measure the collective charges from the heart and the brain, respectively. Every lowly cell has some function that requires glucose (fuel) plus these electrical forces not only to manufacture the enzymes but also to allow them to function.

Not all the known ninety-two elements are essential to the function of the human body. Ninety-eight percent of the human body consists of oxygen (65 percent), carbon (18.5 percent), hydrogen (9.5 percent), and nitrogen (3.3 percent). Even with all those bones and teeth, calcium only accounts for 1.5 percent. The rest of the body consists of boron, chlorine, chromium, cobalt, copper, fluorine, iodine, iron, magnesium, manganese, molybdenum, phosphorus, potassium, selenium, silicon, sodium, sulfur, tin, and zinc.

All of these minerals have important functions in the work of the body's enzymes. Vitamins, amino acids, and specific minerals are used to make the enzymes. The enzymes need a substrate like a cupboard with a constant supply of the proper items in the right concentrations and ratios. (Without chromium insulin cannot make dextrose function. Without iodine thyroxin is worthless. Magnesium is needed for the action of three hundred or so enzymes. Iron, carbon, and nitrogen are required for the hemoglobin molecule. Sodium is required to convert cholesterol to testosterone.)

Oxygen is one of the most electronegative of the ninety-two elements, attracting shared electrons more strongly than $H+$. Carbon bonds to oxygen, hydrogen, nitrogen, sulfur, and chlorine. There are over a million organic (carbon containing) compounds known. Because of the very stable $C = C$ bonds, carbon can make large molecules as its outer shell is only half filled with electrons. With only four outer shell vacancies, carbon can form and build extended molecular structures. Carbon chains can bind together to make long chains as in fatty acids, or to make cyclic compounds such as cholesterol. This unique property of carbon allows for the versatility of living organisms.

Water, H_2O, makes life possible. Cells are 75 to 95 percent water. Most of compounds of the rest of the cell are carbon-based, such as proteins, DNA, and sugars. These are carbon plus H (hydrogen), O (oxygen), N (nitrogen), S (sulfur), and P (phosphorus). Most chemical reactions in the human take place when the reactants are dissolved in water. (E.g., oxygen is dissolved in serum and then bonds to hemoglobin, which carries it from the lungs to the tissues.) Oils will not dissolve in water because water molecules are polar: The strong electrical forces between the water molecules do not allow the penetration of the oil droplets. The function of molecules in the cells are very sensitive to the concentration of the $H+$ and the $OH-$ ions. Buffers, such as the salts mentioned in the electrolyte chapter, and the weak acids, such as carbonic acid, maintain the pH at a slightly alkaline state.

This mini-chemistry lesson is to alert the reader that he/she cannot cheat those cells, those enzymes, those atoms that will become molecules and so facilitate life. We need water and all those elements so that the work of the body will continue. Any symptom means a chemical tilt. We must eat and take supplements to help our bodies perform its maintenance functions.

If we have provided the appropriate vitamins, minerals, amino and fatty acids, the cells are happily doing their jobs. If the cells are happy, then we feel good and have no symptoms. However, can we trust our planet to supply those nutrients we all need? We already know about our topsoil, the devastation of food processing, and overcooked foods.

People all over the world for thousands of years have discovered that certain foods from certain areas have been curative for specific illnesses. Almost two hundred years ago, Alexander von Humboldt noticed that goiter (swollen thyroid gland) was common in the Andean highlands in Colombia, but unheard of in a nearby valley. A French chemist, Jean-Baptiste Boussingault, investigated this apparent discrepancy. In an abandoned mine in that goiter-free valley he found a seepage of brine with the scent of seawater. He noted that the natives drank this brine occasionally. When the mountain people with goiters came to this valley and "took the waters," their goiters disappeared. It was rich in iodine, and I bet it smelled good to those who needed it.

Beginning in 1860 in France and then in the U.S. in 1917 iodine was added to the diets of those living in goiter belts. By 1924 iodized salt became standard. Now, however, most of the iodine comes from dairy products as iodine-containing disinfectants are used by the dairy industry to clean equipment, plus the iodine in the feed of the cows. (Statement by the National Academy of Sciences, 1989.)

Research has discovered the deficiency explaining the not uncommon sexual immaturity of many Eastern Mediterranean men. These men have prepubertal sexual organs and lack of pubic hair at ages of 18 years and older. It is known that zinc is necessary for the development of secondary sexual characteristics and testicular function. If the diet is high in unleavened bread, the low zinc in that food may be chelated (combined) with phytic acid and is unavailable for absorption. Yeast in the manufacture of bread destroys the phytic acid and the zinc becomes available to the ingester.

We are all familiar with the scurvy story of the British sailors before they were given limes and other C-bearing foods by the Royal Navy. Before these scorbutic sailors died of their scurvy, they were thought to be malingerers and were occasionally keelhauled to "bring them around." How many people are dragging around today because they have a deficiency of one sort or another or the cells are not being nourished with the proper atoms and molecules?

I learned in medical school that nutrition had little to do with sickness except for the alcoholic who forgot to eat, the anorectic who would not eat, and the obese person who could not stop eating. The government had stepped in to help us with the National Academy of Sciences' Recommended Daily Allowances (RDA): 40 mg of C, 2 mg of each of the Bs, etc., but on a modern diet it was hard to reach those minimal amounts, because our foods are so nutrient-deficient. Some researchers have defied our government edicts and actually figured out what we were getting on a "good, healthy American diet."

The following tables show how a "well-balanced" diet is not balanced. The man and woman eating the following lists of foods will be unable to get the vitamins and minerals needed to be healthy. Each food is broken down to show the vitamin and mineral content. The totals for each column are shown at the bottom of the page along with the RDA for the "average healthy" man and woman twenty-three to fifty years of age.

A Close Look at a "Balanced Diet"

Changing your chemistry takes time. How do you know what foods you need to balance your chemistry?

By carefully studying the following charts, showing an example of a "balanced diet," it will be easy to see how quickly patterns develop. Even when following a balanced diet patterns of nutritional deficiency will soon emerge.

By continuing to follow established dietary patterns, an individual or an entire family soon develops long-term deficiencies and excesses. Most people repeat basically the same diet over months and years, often extending to generations.

The diet shown below follows what is generally considered a "well-balanced" diet. This is not a diet meant to be followed but is used to demonstrate how a "well-balanced" diet is *not balanced*.

Each food is broken down to show the vitamin and mineral content. Please note, in many cases the portions are much smaller than normally considered a "serving size." There are no snacks, beverages (soft drinks, beer, tea, and so forth) except those with meals.

The nutritional information for each column is totalled for the day at the bottom of the page. Compare these totals against the RDA (broken out separately for "average healthy" men and women between twenty-three and fifty years of age) to see how "a balanced diet" is apt to be insufficient in some areas, and excessive in others.

"A BALANCED DIET:" THE FIRST DAY

Some levels of nutrients are extremely high—note for instance, the excess Vitamin A and Vitamin C—while others, such as

TABLE 9.1
A Balanced Diet, The First Day

	Measure	Weight (g)	Calories	Protein (g)	Fats (g)	Carbohydrates (g)	Water (g)	Vitamin A (IU)	B₁ (Thiamine) (mg)	B₂ (Riboflavin) (mg)	Vitamin B₆ (mg)	Vitamin B₁₂ (mcg)	Vitamin C (mg)	Vitamin D (IU)	Vitamin E (mg)
Breakfast															
Fr. Grapefruit	1 med.	260	108	1.3	.3	25	230	1144	.16	.06	.09	0	105	—	.58
Hot Farina	1 cup	238	131	4.1	.2	26	204	0	.17	.1	.05	0	0	0	—
Pancake	1 (4″)	45	104	3.2	3.2	15.3	22.5	54	.08	.1	—	—	t	—	—
Maple Syrup	1 tbsp.	20	50	0	0	13	6.6	0	—	—	—	—	0	—	—
Butter	1 tbsp.	14	100	.1	11.2	.1	2.2	462	—	—	t	t	0	13	.14
Coffee, Black	1 cup	230	2	.3	.1	.8	226	0	.01	.01	t	t	0	0	—
Milk, Whole	1 cup	244	159	8.5	8.8	12	213	354	.07	.42	.09	.98	2.44	100	.1
Lunch															
Baked Ham	4 oz.	113	327	23.75	25	0	60.75	0	.533	2.04	.508	.8	0	0	1.8
Bak. Sweet Pot.	1 sm.	100	141	2.1	.5	32.5	64	8100	.09	.07	.218	0	22	—	—
Broccoli	1 cup	150	39	4.6	.4	6.7	137	3750	.135	.3	.26	0	135	—	—
Waldorf Salad	1 cup	200	180	2.5	10	21	—	475	.11	.09	—	—	7	—	—
Roll, Whole Wh.	1 med.	40	103	4	1.1	19.5	12.8	t	.14	.05	—	t	t	—	—
Butter	1 tbsp.	14	100	.1	11.2	.1	2.2	462	—	—	t	t	0	13	.14
Ice Cream	1 av.	80	188	4	7.5	24	—	302	.04	.17	—	—	0	0	—
Milk, Whole	1 cup	244	159	8.5	8.8	12	213	354	.07	.42	.09	.98	2.44	100	.1
Dinner															
Ham Sandwich	1 av.	81	281	11	15	24	—	30	.28	.14	—	—	2	—	—
Raw Carrot St.	1 lg.	100	42	1.1	.2	9.7	88	11000	.06	.05	.15	0	8	—	.11
Fruit Cup	1 cup	256	195	1	.3	47	204	358	.05	.03	.085	0	5.12	—	—
Sugar Cookie	1 lge.	8	36	.5	1.3	5.4	.6	6	.001	.01	—	—	0	—	—
Milk, Whole	1 cup	244	159	8.5	8.8	12	213	354	.07	.42	.09	.98	2.44	100	.1
Totals															
Food total			2604	89	114	306	1900	27205	2.069	4.5	1.6	3.74	291	326	3.07
R.D.A. Men 23–50			2600	56	87	390		5000	1.2	1.5	2	3	45	400	15
R.D.A. Women 23–50			2000	46	66	300		4000	1	1.2	2	3	45	400	12

	Measure	Biotin (mcg)	Choline (mg)	Calcium (mg)	Folic Acid (mg)	Inositol (g)	Iron (mg)	Magnesium (mg)	Niacin (mg)	Pantothenic Acid (mg)	Potassium (mg)	Iodine (mg)	Phosphorus (mg)	Sodium (mg)
Breakfast														
Fr. Grapefruit	1 med.	78	—	46	.01	.47	1.14	31.2	.57	.07	385	—	46	2.9
Hot Farina	1 cup	—	—	183	—	—	15	9.5	1.2	—	31	—	143	447
Pancake	1 (4")	—	—	45	—	—	.6	11	.6	—	55	—	63	191
Maple Syrup	1 tbsp.	—	—	21	—	—	.24	—	0	—	35	—	1.6	2
Butter	1 tbsp.	—	.7	2.8	—	—	0	1.9	—	—	3	.46	2	138
Coffee, Black	1 cup	—	—	4.6	—	—	.23	15.4	.9	.01	83	—	5	2.3
Milk, Whole	1 cup	—	36.6	287	.002	.03	t	37	.24	.75	346	—	226	122
Lunch														
Baked Ham	4 oz.	5.68	137.5	10	.0025	.035	2.95	22.65	.408	.9	376	—	194.8	813
Bak. Sweet Pot.	1 sm.	4.3	11.5	40	.015	.07	.9	31	.7	.82	300	—	58	12
Broccoli	1 cup	3.1	—	132	.08	—	1.2	36	1.2	1.9	401	—	93	15
Waldorf Salad	1 cup	—	—	43	—	—	1.1	46	.6	—	—	—	64	—
Roll, Whole Wh.	1 med.	—	—	42	—	—	.96	—	1.2	—	117	—	112	226
Butter	1 tbsp.	—	.7	2.8	—	—	0	1.9	—	—	3	.46	2	138
Ice Cream	1 av.	—	—	108	.002	—	1.8	5.2	.04	.07	152	—	102	69
Milk, Whole	1 cup	—	36.6	287	.002	.03	t	37	.24	.75	346	—	226	122
Dinner														
Ham Sandwich	1 av.	2.5	13.4	40	—	—	1.7	—	2.3	—	—	—	93	—
Raw Carrot St.	1 lg.	—	—	37	.008	.05	.7	23	.6	.28	341	—	36	47
Fruit Cup	1 cup	—	—	23	—	—	1.02	17.9	1.02	—	412	—	31	13
Sugar Cookie	1 lge.	—	—	6.2	—	—	.11	—	.02	—	6	—	8.2	13
Milk, Whole	1 cup	—	36.6	287	.002	.03	t	37	.24	.75	346	—	226	122
Totals														
Food total		94	274	1647	.124	.72	30	364	12	6.3	3738	.92	1733	2495
R.D.A. Men 23–50		150–300	500–900	800	.4	1000	10	350	16	5–10	1950–5850	110	800	2300–6900
R.D.A. Women 23–50		150–300	500–900	800	.4	1000	18	300	13	5–10	1950–5850	100	800	2300–6900

TABLE 9.2
A Balanced Diet, The Second Day

	Measure	Weight (g)	Calories	Protein (g)	Fats (g)	Carbohydrates (g)	Water (g)	Vitamin A (IU)	(Thiamine) B_1 (mg)	(Riboflavin) B_2 (mg)	Vitamin B_6 (mg)	Vitamin B_{12} (mcg)	Vitamin C (mg)	Vitamin D (IU)	Vitamin E (mg)
Breakfast															
Sliced Orange	1 med.	180	88	1.8	.4	20	154	360	.18	.05	.18	0	90	0	.43
Cr. of Wheat	1 cup	200	134	4.5	.4	28	175	.11	.07	—	.045	—	—	50	.05
Milk, Whole	½ cup	122	79	4.25	4.4	6	106.5	177	.035	.21	—	.49	1.22	0	—
Sugar	1 tsp.	12	46	0	0	12	—	0	0	—	—	—	—	—	—
Toast, Whole Wh.	1 sl.	19	55	2.4	.6	11	5.6	t	.04	.02	—	—	t	—	—
Butter	1 tbsp.	14	100	.1	11.2	.1	2.2	462	t	.01	—	—	—	13	.14
Jelly	1 tbsp.	20	55	t	t	14	5.8	2	.01	.01	—	0	.8	0	—
Coffee, Black	1 cup	230	2	.3	.1	.8	226	0	t	—	—	0	0	—	—
Lunch															
Tomato Soup w/Water	1 cup	240	86	1.9	2.4	15	217	1176	.1	.25	—	—	15	—	—
Gr. Cheese Sand. w/American Ch.	1 av.	68	227	10.5	8.54	24.5	11.1	342	.106	.22	.02	.2	0	—	—
Sweet Pickle	1 med.	100	146	.7	.4	36.5	6.1	90	t	.02	—	—	6	—	—
Can. Apricots	1 cup	250	215	1.5	.2	53	193	4350	.05	.05	.135	—	10	—	—
Choc. Chip Cook.	1 med.	9	46	.5	2.7	5.3	.3	10	.01	.01	.09	—	t	—	—
Milk, Whole	1 cup	244	159	8.5	8.8	12	213	354	.07	.42	.09	.98	2.44	100	.1
Dinner															
Fried Liver	4 oz.	113	263	30	12	6	63.5	60475	.3	4.73	.95	—	30.5	38.5	.73
Froz. Mix. Veg.	1 cup	234	150	7.5	.7	31.4	193	1158	.28	.16	.29	—	18.7	—	.04
Broiled Potato	1 med.	100	76	2.1	.1	17.1	80	t	.09	.04	.174	—	16	—	—
Cole Slaw	1 cup	120	173	1.6	16.8	5.8	95	192	.06	.06	.02	—	34.8	—	.23
Bread, En. White	1 sl.	23	62	2	.7	12	8.2	t	.06	.05	t	—	t	—	—
Butter	1 tbsp.	14	100	.1	11.2	.1	2.2	462	—	—	—	t	0	13	.14
Choc. Pudding	1 cup	248	367	7.7	12	64	163	372	.05	.35	—	—	0	—	—
Totals															
Food total		2629		87.75	94.1	374.6	1976	69640	1.511	6.66	1.914	1.67	225.6	215	1.86
R.D.A. Men 23–50		2600		56	87	390		5000	1.2	1.5	2	3	45	400	15
R.D.A. Women 23–50		2000		46	66	300		4000	1	1.2	2	3	45	400	12

	Measure	Biotin (mcg)	Choline (mg)	Calcium (mg)	Folic Acid (mg)	Inositol (g)	Iron (mg)	Magnesium (mg)	Niacin (mg)	Pantothenic Acid (mg)	Potassium (mg)	Iodine (mg)	Phosphorus (mg)	Sodium (mg)
Breakfast														
Sliced Orange	1 med.	t	—	74	.01	.38	.72	19.8	.72	.45	360	—	36	1.8
Cr. of Wheat	1 cup	—	—	99	—	—	9	—	.3	—	—	—	124	—
Milk, Whole	½ cup	—	18.3	143.5	.001	.015	—	18.5	.12	.038	173	—	113	6.1
Sugar	1 tsp.	—	—	.6	—	—	.01	t	0	—	t	—	.1	.1
Toast, Whole Wh.	1 sl.	—	—	22	.01	.01	.5	18	.6	—	62	—	52	119
Butter	1 tbsp.	—	.7	2.8	—	—	0	1.9	—	—	3	—	2	138
Jelly	1 tbsp.	—	—	4.2	—	—	.3	1	.04	—	15	.46	1.4	3.4
Coffee, Black	1 cup	—	—	4.6	—	—	.23	15.4	.9	.01	83	—	5	2.3
Lunch														
Tomato Soup w/Water	1 cup	—	—	14	—	—	.72	22	1.23	—	226	—	34	1034
Gr. Cheese Sand. w/American Ch.	1 av.	1.3	—	235	.003	—	1.41	23	.56	.13	70	—	262	554
Sweet Pickle	1 med.	—	—	12	—	—	1.2	1	t	—	—	—	16	—
Can. Apricots	1 cup	—	—	28	.015	—	.75	17.5	t	.23	585	—	38	2.5
Choc. Chip Cook.	1 med.	—	—	3.1	—	—	.2	—	.08	—	11	—	8.9	31
Milk, Whole	1 cup	—	36.6	287	.002	.03	t	37	.24	.75	346	—	226	122
Dinner														
Fried Liver	4 oz.	112.5	577.5	12.25	.333	.058	8.91	20.5	18.68	8.73	430.3	—	477.3	208.5
Froz. Mix. Veg.	1 cup	—	—	58.5	.04	.03	3	—	2.6	.73	447	—	147	124
Boiled Potato	1 med.	—	29	7	.007	—	.6	—	1.5	.4	407	—	53	3
Cole Slaw	1 cup	—	—	3.48	—	—	.48	5	.36	—	239	—	34.8	144
Bread, En. White	1 sl.	—	—	19	.003	—	.58	1.9	.55	.1	24	—	22	177
Butter	1 tbsp.	.2	.7	2.8	—	—	0	—	—	—	3	.46	2	138
Choc. Pudding	1 cup	—	—	238	—	—	1.24	—	.25	—	424	—	243	139
Totals														
Food total		114	662.8	1271	.424	.523	29.85	202.5	28.73	11.57	3908	.92	1829	2888
R.D.A. Men 23–50		150–300	500–900	800	.4	1000	10	350	16	5–10	1950–5850	110	800	2300–6900
R.D.A. Women 23–50		150–300	500–900	800	.4	1000	18	300	13	5–10	1950–5850	100	800	2300–6900

TABLE 9.3
A Balanced Diet, The Third Day

	Measure	Weight (g)	Calories	Protein (g)	Fats (g)	Carbohydrates (g)	Water (g)	Vitamin A (IU)	(Thiamine) B_1 (mg)	(Riboflavin) B_2 (mg)	Vitamin B_6 (mg)	Vitamin B_{12} (mcg)	Vitamin C (mg)	Vitamin D (IU)	Vitamin E (mg)
Breakfast															
Fr. Grapefruit	1 med.	260	108	1.3	.3	25	230	1144	.16	.06	.09	0	105	—	.58
Cr. of Rice	¾ c.	—	120	2	0	26	—	t	—	t	—	—	t	—	—
French Toast	1 sl.	65	183	5.5	12	14	—	.09	.16	—	—	—	t	—	—
Coffee, Black	1 cup	230	2	.3	.1	.8	226	0	.01	.01	t	0	0	0	—
Milk, Whole	1 cup	244	159	8.5	8.8	12	213	354	.07	.42	.09	.98	2.44	100	.1
Lunch															
Omelet	1 med.	64	116	7.6	8.3	1.5	46	691	.05	.18	—	—	0	31	—
Tomato Aspic Salad	1 sq.	106	43	1.132	—	10.6	102.6	407	.029	.015	.104	—	10.37	—	—
Bread, Rye	1 sl.	23	56	2.1	.3	12	8.2	0	.04	.02	.023	0	0	—	—
Fresh Pear	1 med.	182	111	1.3	.7	27.8	151	36	.04	.08	.034	0	7.28	—	—
Choc. Milk w/Skim milk	1 cup	290	220	9.6	6.7	32	240	232	.12	.46	.13	.4	2.5	—	—
Dinner															
Roast Pork Chops	2½ oz.	90	338	20.4	.2	0	40.8	0	.46	.208	.434	—	0	0	.64
Scallop. Pot. Ch.	1 cup	133	193	7.1	10.5	18.1	95	426	.08	.16	—	—	13.3	—	—
Apple Sauce	1 cup	300	273	.6	.3	71.4	227	120	.06	.03	.05	0	3	—	—
Can. Peas	1 cup	100	66	3.5	.3	12.5	82.6	450	.09	.05	.08	0	9	—	.02
Bread, Whole Wht	1 sl.	23	55	2.1	.6	11	8.4	t	.07	.02	—	0	t	—	—
Choc. Cake	1 svg.	10	38	.3	1.4	6.7	1.4	21	.002	.01	—	0	t	.1	—
Coffee, Black	1 cup	230	2	.3	.1	.8	226	0	.01	.01	t	0	0	0	—
Milk, Whole	1 cup	244	159	8.5	8.8	12	213	354	.07	.42	.09	.98	2.44	100	.1
Totals															
Food total			2122	80.13	59.4	268.2	2111	4235	1.521	2.153	1.125	2.36	155.6	231	1.44
R.D.A. Men 23–50			2600	56	87	390		5000	1.2	1.5	2	3	45	400	15
R.D.A. Women 23–50			2000	46	66	300		4000	1	1.2	2	3	45	400	12

	Measure	Biotin (mcg)	Choline (mg)	Calcium (mg)	Folic Acid (mg)	Inositol (g)	Iron (mg)	Magnesium (mg)	Niacin (mg)	Pantothenic Acid (mg)	Potassium (mg)	Iodine (mg)	Phosphorus (mg)	Sodium (mg)
Breakfast														
Fr. Grapefruit	1 med.	78	—	46	.01	.47	1.14	31.2	.57	.07	385	—	46	2.9
Cr. of Rice	¾ C.	—	—	t	—	—	—	—	—	—	—	—	—	10
French Toast	1 sl.	—	—	77	—	—	.9	16	.5	—	—	—	94	—
Coffee, Black	1 cup	—	—	4.6	—	—	.23	15.4	.9	.01	83	—	5	2.3
Milk, Whole	1 cup	—	36.6	287	.002	.03	t	37	.24	.75	346	—	226	122
Lunch														
Omelet	1 med.	—	—	51	—	—	1.1	7	.1	—	93	—	121	164
Tomato Aspic Salad	1 sq.	—	—	8.35	.004	—	.49	8.42	.416	.145	144.5	1	10.81	603
Bread, Rye	1 sl.	—	—	17	.004	.32	.37	10	.1	—	33	—	34	128
Fresh Pear	1 med.	t	—	15	—	—	.6	12.7	.18	.13	237	—	20	3.6
Choc. Milk w/Skim milk	1 cup	11.4	38	313	.003	—	.58	—	.5	1.6	411	—	263	133
Dinner														
Roast Pork Chops	2½ oz.	4.72	69.8	9.06	.002	.04	2.6	24.4	4.4	.398	514.6	—	210.2	54.4
Scallop Pot. Ch.	1 cup	—	—	169	—	—	.67	—	1.2	—	407	—	162	595
Apple Sauce	1 cup	—	—	12	.01	t	1.5	15	.9	.15	195	—	15	6
Can. Peas	1 cup	—	—	20	.01	—	1.7	20	.64	.18	96	—	66	236
Bread, Whole Wht.	1 sl.	.4	—	19	—	.01	.53	18	.02	—	59	—	58	122
Choc. Cake	1 svg.	—	—	6	—	—	.1	15.4	.9	.01	20	—	11	6
Coffee, Black	1 cup	—	—	4.6	—	—	.23	37	.9	—	83	—	5	2.3
Milk, Whole	1 cup	—	36.6	287	.002	.03	t	129.8	.24	.75	346	—	226	122
Totals														
Food total		94.42	181.4	1058	.047	.9	12.74	268	11.81	4.2	3453	1	1573	2303
R.D.A. Men 23–50		150–300	500–900	800	.4	1000	10	350	16	5–10	1950–5850	110	800	2300–6900
R.D.A. Women 23–50		150–300	500–900	800	.4	1000	18	300	13	5–10	1950–5850	100	800	2300–6900

Vitamin E, are extremely low. These values vary day to day, being high on one day and low the next. Others remain constantly high or low. These sheets demonstrate the lack of merit in a "well-balanced" diet.

"A BALANCED DIET:" THE SECOND DAY

We tend to eat the same diet over the years, therefore medical problems tend to get progressively worse. Special diets are used to regulate diseases such as: diabetes, arthritis, heart disease, and hypoglycemia. Specific diets such as these tend to help one specific problem and ignore basic nutrition, creating new problems. Note the excess vitamin A, B_2, and C, and deficiency of vitamins E, B_{12}, D, biotin, and magnesium.

"A BALANCED DIET:" THE THIRD DAY

Following a "balanced diet," you'll note the inconsistency of the nutrient levels. Research shows that such a diet cannot provide balanced nutrition, even according to the RDA standards. Note that some of the levels are high day after day, compounding the imbalance; vitamin C is the only nutrient consistently in excess, while the majority of the others are very deficient. Adding these excesses and deficiencies over time, the ingester will end up with a disease sooner or later.

Who Needs Vitamins and Minerals?

Just a decade ago, Arthur Sackler, M.D., columnist for the *Medical Tribune*, pointed out that about half of the population in the U.S. had diagnosable illnesses: there are ten million alcoholics, thirty-five million with allergies, thirty million with arthritis, twelve million diabetics, and twenty-five million hypertensives. These were but the diagnosed ones and did not include those with chronic backaches, depression, fatigue, migraines, intestinal pathology, kidney failure, emphysema, multiple sclerosis, schizophrenia, cancer, premenstrual syndrome, glaucoma, cataracts, and genetic malformations. He did not even include the geriatric group who are suffering from a variety of problems related to age and malabsorption associated with defective stomach acid production. (This all adds up to more than our population as many people have two or three of the above problems simultaneously.)

Without stretching credulity too much we can find chemical deviations and nutritional deficiencies in all these conditions—some more, some less—that either allowed the disease to become manifest or showed up after the disease was established. It is astounding that our government cannot accept the nutritional facts of our sick society. If our officials would just proscribe the use of sugar and bleached grains, health costs could be cut in half.

There is no doubt that we are being cheated because of the erosion of the topsoil, the removal of essential nutrients by food manufacturers to maintain shelf life, and the loss of vitamins and minerals from cooking. It seems logical to any of us who have studied nutrition that the rise in the incidence of degenerative disease is exactly related to the depletion of the nutrients in the foods that are swallowed.

We have discovered that the diets of primitive people led to healthy lives free of heart attacks, high blood pressure, strokes, constipation, diverticulosis, hiatal hernia, and diabetes. The facts are there and obvious. We need our government to take some leadership to at least *encourage* a healthy lifestyle. The government has funded in-depth studies but it does not seem to act upon its findings. (E.g., vitamin A levels have been found to be 40 percent below the acceptable levels in a national survey a few years ago.)

It appears, then, that even if we do lead a stressless life, eat fresh foods from our backyard—cooked minimally, breathe mountain-fresh air, drink clear, distilled water, we may not achieve health and vigor, because we must rely on the earth, which apparently has slipped a little from perfection since it was put together eons ago. Most of that is man-made, but some of it is just the natural course of aging. The aging earth is getting more alkaline, and, as a consequence, so are we.

Darwin came to the general conclusion that living things adapt to changes in their environments and the strengths or weaknesses that change brings determines the result. Our environment has changed in the last few decades, and it may be that our increased rate of sickness, cancer, delinquency, and mental illness is our ''unique'' way of adapting.

Kitkoski has been able to determine how farming has altered the levels of nitrogen elements in the blood and pushed chemistry to the alkaline side. Farmers to the west and southwest of Spokane use nitrogen fertilizer to grow wheat. Of the amount applied, 17 percent stays in the soil to be utilized by the plant, the remaining nitrogen evaporates into the atmosphere. Most of the year the prevailing winds carry the nitrogen-laden air to Spokane. Since nitrogen is heavier than oxygen, it settles over and around Spokane. When the sun shines on excess nitrogen it causes oxidation of the nitrogen to nitrates and nitrites, which settle on the city as they are heavy molecules. If there is not enough ventilation, normal aeration for animals, plants, and humans will cause sickness. And does. The rains come and wash the nitrates into the soil. Burning garbage to the west and south of Spokane will aggravate the pollution problem. The oxygen needed to burn the garbage is already in short supply because oxygen is now bound to the nitrogen. When this air gets to Spokane the carbon from industry, burning, and car exhausts cannot be oxidized sufficiently. No wonder that Spokane has the distinction of being one of the U.S. cites with a high rate of carbon monoxide in the air.

Everything we do to correct one problem appears to create two or three other problems. We are all tied together like a web (see page 233).

Phosphates in the lakes were promoting the growth of algae, so hundreds of tons of aluminum were then dumped into the lakes to tie up the phosphates. This alum (potassium aluminum sulfate), however, creates a new problem: alkalinity. This water eventually gets to the oceans. Could this alum be poisoning the whales who may be beaching themselves because they have a type of whale-Alzheimer's?

The waste material from the extraction of aluminum from its ore is called magnasite. Farmers use this as fertilizer not realizing that the seasonal changes, soil moisture, sunlight, rain, and heat oxidizes these chemicals. The magnesium, calcium, sulfur, and zinc in this residuum, catalyzed by the weather, creates carbon monoxide as a byproduct. The nitrogen-fixing bacteria in the soil need CO_2, not CO, to make proper plants. Farmers need to use crops that are able to fix nitrogen to the roots, like alfalfa.

Everything that is added or removed affects our food chain by creating excesses and deficiencies leading to the diseases we acquire. In areas where the nitrates in the soil are excessive, the blood tests of the people eating those locally grown foods has been slowly changing over the last few decades. The blood urea nitrogen (BUN) has increased as have the iron levels. The soil alkalinity has been increasing over the years, and, as a consequence, in the bodies of the people who eat foods grown in that soil.

The fluorocarbons, pesticides, and acid rain affect the ozone layer, killing trees and fish. But just as importantly, the byproducts of manufacturing are changing the topsoil. When the ratios of the mineral and the acid/base balance is shifted, the plants are different. The amount of abuse grows with the number of farmers. The ratios are changed enough to change even the climate. Nitrogen (80 percent of the air) and hydrogen are most abused. The form of the nitrogen has been changed to make fertilizers, pesticides, herbicides, and food preservative.

The plant/soil/animal system is affected when we change the pH. Alteration of soil acidity kills the nitrogen-fixing bacteria. New bacteria are created. The rain washes the nitrates out of the air, which changes the plants; they become protein-deficient due to lack of usable nitrogen. The cattle get sick. They are given antibiotics, which alter their manure. The bacteria needed to break down the manure to release nitrogen to nourish the plants is not available. The unhealthy plants die allowing the weeds to take over the pasture. These weeds are not proper nutrition for cattle. Because of poor nutrition, the cattle are sold as a lower grade meat. This meat has a higher percentage of nitrates because of the plants. (You could substitute the human being for the cattle in the above scenario and recreate an accurate paradigm of what is happening all over.) The soil, the plants, the animals, and the humans all suffer.

Linus Pauling has this to say: "Life is the cumulative product of interaction among the many kinds of chemical substances that make up the cells of an organism."

10

Normal Human Chemistry: Analysis of the Blood Tests

You don't have to be a rocket scientist to figure out what your blood tests mean. The tests establish the scientific credibility of the theme of this book: Your blood chemistry proves that you may trust your senses of taste and smell to determine your nutritional needs. The correlation among the levels of the elements, enzymes, and chemicals in the blood and the senses is real, palpable, and reproducible. Your symptoms are a clue that something is amiss. The blood test defines that imbalance.

First you have to have the blood test results in your hand. Ask your doctor, of course, to order the following tests to be done on your blood (The blood is to be drawn after you have fasted overnight—usually for twelve hours; water is allowed. When the blood is drawn, the fist should not be clenched as it will produce a falsely high potassium level.): The CBC (complete blood count), the diff (the percents of the different types of white cells), the serum iron, and the 24 chemical screen (includes fasting glucose, BUN, creatinine, sodium, potassium, chloride, CO_2, uric acid, calcium, phosphorus, total protein, albumin, cholesterol, triglycerides, GGT, SGOT, SGPT, LDH, alkaline phosphatase, total bilirubin, including direct and indirect).

The printout shows your values and the values the laboratory considers within the "normal range." This normal range is taken from the values of thousands of clients, sick or well. They remove the readings of those that are at the top 5 percent and the bottom 5 percent. The remaining 90 percent are considered by the lab as the usual and customary.

Your doctor is concerned only if any of your test scores fall outside the 90 percent range. Are they are too high or too low? The method used by the Life Balances program described in this book is the deviation from the mean, the value that is halfway between the high and the low inside that normal range. (E.g.: the range for calcium is usually 8.5 to 10.5 mg per deciliter. The mean is 9.5.)

The following is true for all the values: If only one test is off from the mean by a small percent, it is not a serious problem of and by itself. If in many tests the values are slightly above or below the mean, there might be a serious overload or a major deficiency. Either way, the summation of the deviant scores indicates that a problem is present or soon to appear. Notice how far off you are from the mean. The following is a description of what each test indicates and what diseases and conditions may be responsible for significant highs and lows. If a "normal" person has fasted for twelve hours before the blood was drawn, the result would fall in the *usual* range indicated below. The lab does not flag any value in that range as abnormal. The *optimal* range is closer to health and the *mean* would be as close to perfect as one can get.

FASTING GLUCOSE

Glucose is blood sugar, the primary source of energy for most cells. It is regulated by inhibitors and stimulators (insulin and glucagon from the pancreas, thyroid hormone, liver enzymes, and adrenal hormones). Best drawn after a twelve-hour fast. Insulin lowers and glucagon raises the sugar level. The liver converts other sugars, lactic acid, proteins, and fats into glucose.

- *Usual:* 65 to 110 mg/dl
- *Optimum:* 75 to 100 mg/dl
- *Mean:* 87.5 mg/dl

It may be elevated in diabetes, liver disease, obesity, hyperthyroidism, stress, pancreatitis, steroid drugs, and oral contraceptives or a meal high in sugar and starches one to four hours before the blood was drawn. Food sensitivities make the blood sugar rise in some people to the point that they may be erroneously diagnosed as being diabetic. It may be below normal if there is excess insulin, liver disease, malabsorption, hypothyroidism, or alcoholism. This indicates an oversupply of suppressors or that the stimulators are weakened.

BUN

The blood urea nitrogen is the nitrogen part of urea, the end product of protein breakdown. Protein foods are broken down to amino acids. When these are metabolized, the remaining nitrogen becomes a part of urea. Urea is formed in the liver and excreted by the kidneys.

- *Usual:* 8 to 23 mg/dl
- *Optimum:* 12 to 19 mg/dl
- *Mean:* 15.5 mg/dl

A slight increase of BUN indicates an excessive protein intake. Or it may be elevated if there is kidney damage, strenuous exercise, poor fluid intake, intestinal bleeding, the intake of certain drugs, or heart failure. If protein intake is limited to 10 to 15 percent of the total calories, a high BUN level can be reduced—if the kidneys are working properly. Elevated BUN may indicate liver or thyroid inactivity. It might be lower because of a low-protein diet, malnutrition, poor absorption, liver damage, or pregnancy. It also may indicate pancreas or adrenal inactivity, or any wasting disease.

CREATININE

This is a waste product of muscle metabolism. The level is a reflection of muscle metabolism and is proportional to the muscle mass. When protein digestion is impaired, muscles break down to supply amino acids.

- *Usual:* male: 0.8 to 1.4 mg/dl
  female: 0.6 to 1.2 mg/dl
- *Optimum:* 0.9 to 1.3 mg/dl
- *Mean:* 1.1 mg/dl

The kidneys excrete creatinine so the level is elevated if kidney disease is present, muscle degeneration, or by the use of any drug that would hurt kidney function. It is lower in some forms of kidney damage, protein starvation, impaired protein digestion, liver disease, or pregnancy.

BUN/CREATININE RATIO

If the ratio is very high then too much BUN is being formed. If the ratio is very low, then the creatinine is not being cleared through the kidneys. It is a sensitive measurement of kidney and liver function, and protein ingestion and metabolism.

- *Usual:* 6 to 30
- *Optimum:* 10 to 26
- *Mean:* 18

SODIUM

Sodium is one of the several electrolytes. It is necessary for the maintenance of blood pressure, the acid-base balance, production of digestive fluids, and nerve function. It controls viscosity and ionic balance of blood, muscle function, and is necessary for growth and longevity. Its level is regulated by the kidneys and the adrenal glands.

- *Usual:* 135 to 148 mEq/L
- *Optimum:* 137 to 143 mEq/L
- *Mean:* 141.5 mEq/L

It may be above normal due to a high-salt diet (foods always salted during cooking and after serving; processed foods are salty). Elevated sodium-levels are associated with hypertension, anemia, kidney, and liver diseases. It leads to alkalinity. Fluid retention is often associated with a high sodium level in the blood. It may be low due to ingestion of boiled foods, excessive water intake, vegetarian diet, diarrhea, and kidney failure. A low level is associated with an acidic condition.

POTASSIUM

The major intracellular cation (electrolyte carrying a positive charge) it tends to alkalinize the blood. It maintains cellular osmotic balance, and is involved with the acid-base balance. It is needed for the proper electrical conduction in nerves and muscles, especially for the heart. Its levels are regulated by adrenal hormones, glucose, and sodium. It is elevated when tissue decomposes. It regulates enzymes, especially those involved with carbohydrate metabolism.

- *Usual:* 3.4 to 5.2 mEq/L
- *Optimum:* 3.6 to 5 mEq/L
- *Mean:* 4.3 mEq/L

Kidney disease, diabetes, burns, shock, myocardial infarction, slow heart beat, and respiratory diseases are associated with a high potassium level in the blood. It reads low when there is a loss of body fluids as in diarrhea, and a chronic use of diuretics, or by kidney disease, malnutrition, excess insulin, stress, high-meat/low-vegetable diet. Low potassium is often associated with a rapid heart beat.

CHLORIDE

This is an acidifying electrolyte. It helps to maintain the balance between acid and alkaline levels. A high level of chloride makes the blood more acidic. It reflects fluid exchange across cell membranes and it helps to regulate blood pressure, blood volume, and the osmotic pressure of the blood. It is needed for hydrochloric acid production in the stomach.

- *Usual:* 95 to 109 mEq/L
- *Optimum:* 98 to 107 mEq/L
- *Mean:* 102 mEq/L

It may be elevated with acidosis, renal failure, severe dehydration, and hyperventilation. It could be low because of prolonged vomiting, excess fluid retention, inadequate salt intake, diarrhea, excessive sweating replaced only with water, kidney disease, and starvation. People carrying a low level of chloride are more likely to have dilated pupils, scaly skin, indigestion, belching, and intestinal gas, and will suffer from the heat and tend to hyperventilate.

CARBON DIOXIDE (CO_2)

CO_2 is a reflection of the respiratory exchange of carbon dioxide in the lungs and is part of the bicarbonate buffer system. It is one end product of food metabolism. The body functions best at a slightly alkaline level. CO_2 is acidic.

- *Usual:* 22 to 29 mEq/L
- *Optimum:* 23 to 28 mEq/L
- *Mean:* 25.5 mEq/L

It might be up because of severe vomiting, hypoventilation (not breathing deeply enough to exhale CO_2) as in emphysema. Cortisone and diuretic therapy also will elevate the level. Low CO_2 scores are due to starvation, uremia, and respiratory alkalosis, but may be seen in metabolic acidosis (excessive deep breathing due to diabetic acidosis, aspirin ingestion, or alcoholism), hysteria and anxiety (causing hyperventilation), diarrhea, central nervous system disease, vegan vegetarianism, and poor liver function.

URIC ACID

The end product of purine metabolism, uric acid is a normal constituent of the blood. Purines come from cell nuclei (foods high in purines are liver, kidneys, sweetbreads). It is excreted in the urine.

- *Usual:* male: 3.7 to 7.6 mg/dl
  female: 2.5 to 6.2 mg/dl
- *Optimum*: male: 4.5 to 7 mg/dl;
  female: 3 to 5.5 mg/dl
- *Mean*: male: 5.65 mg/dl;
  female: 4.35 mg/dl

A high level usually is usually associated with gout, but kidney disease, infections, excess alcohol or protein ingestion, and toxemia of pregnancy will raise the level. It may be up if there is poor alkaline kidney elimination. A low protein diet, kidney disease, liver atrophy, and malabsorption might result in a low level. An overly acid kidney eliminates uric acid faster than it is being manufactured.

CALCIUM

Calcium is found in teeth and bones. It is needed for coagulation of blood, for the action of many enzymes, regulation of nerves and muscles and is an indicator of protein and fat digestion and absorption. It helps to regulate cell wall permeability. Calcium moves in and out of teeth and bones as needed to maintain the proper blood calcium level; teeth and bones act as calcium reservoirs. If the blood level is low, the parathyroid gland hormone pulls calcium out of the bones to keep the level at the optimum. It is absorbed as the free ion form. The kidneys will control some of the loss ·ia the urine. It is very sensitive to hormonal activity (parathyroid glands, thyroid gland, vitamin D, adrenal steroids), metabolic changes, alkalinity/acidity ratio, and phosphorus. A high-protein diet raises the phosphorus level; this stimulates the secretion of the parathyroid hormone, which pulls the calcium from the bones to maintain the optimal calcium/phosphorus ratio.

- *Usual:* 8.5 to 10.5 mg/dl
- *Optimum:* 9.0 to 10 mg/dl
- *Mean:* 9.5 mg/dl

Elevated levels are found in hyperparathyroidism, hyperthyroidism, with some bone tumors, or excess vitamin D or calcium intake as in antacids, such as calcium carbonate. It might be low due to malnutrition, senescence, kidney dysfunction, hormone imbalance, hypoparathyroidism, tetany, osteoporosis, vitamin D deficiency, and stress. Some symptoms might be paresthesias, hyperirritability, muscle cramps, laryngospasm, convulsions.

PHOSPHORUS

Abundant in all cells and in most tissues, phosphorus is directly related to calcium metabolism. It is needed as a part of energy bonds for carbohydrate metabolism. It is part of the cell wall (phospholipids). It is needed for buffering, calcium transport, and osmotic pressure.

- *Usual*: 2.5 to 4.5 mg/dl
- *Optimum*: 3 to 4 mg/dl
- *Mean*: 3.5 mg/dl

High levels are associated with an alkaline digestive tract due to low hydrochloric acid in the stomach. It is elevated if there is kidney disease, hypoparathyroidism, rapid bone growth, diabetes, excess vitamin D, and liver disease. Low levels are noted if the body is in a hyperacidic condition. It is also low in hyperparathyroidism, vitamin D deficiency, alcoholism, liver disease, and malabsorption. It might be low in a vegetarian diet or a diet high in calcium, iron, and magnesium. Because phosphorus is found in all foods, a deficiency is rare. It may be low in cases of growth retardation, pregnancy, and lactation.

TOTAL PROTEIN

This is the sum of the albumin and the globulin in the blood. They are manufactured in the liver from amino acids in the diet and from the breakdown of protein tissues.

- *Usual:* 6 to 7.7 grams/dl
- *Optimum:* 6.4 to 7.3 grams/dl
- *Mean:* 6.85 grams/dl

ALBUMIN

A protein manufactured by the liver from the amino acids taken in through the diet, albumin is closely correlated with the protein adequacy of the diet. It controls fluid retention (edema) because of the osmotic pressure it maintains, nutrient transport (bilirubin, fatty acids, hormones, vitamins, minerals), and waste removal.

- *Usual:* 3.5 to 5 grams/dl
- *Optimum:* 3.75 to 4.75 grams/dl
- *Mean:* 4.25 grams/dl

It is above the mean if dehydration, shock, multiple myeloma, or liver disease are present. It is lower if the diet is inadequate in protein intake, low viscosity of blood, glomerulonephritis, loss due to diarrhea, hemorrhage, or gastric disorders, fever, infection or malignancy, impaired synthesis due to liver disease, increased need in pregnancy, lactation, or recovery from a disease.

GLOBULIN

A larger protein than albumin, globulin is formed in the liver and is the carrier of some hormones, lipids, and metals. The gamma portion is part of the immune system: the antibodies. Special tests for A, G, M, and E globulins are necessary for the evaluation of patients with allergies or susceptibility to infections.

- *Usual:* 1.6 to 4 grams/dl
- *Optimum:* 2.1 to 3.5 grams/dl
- *Mean:* 2.8 grams/dl

It is elevated in chronic infections, chronic liver disease, rheumatoid arthritis, myeloma, and lupus. It is lower in some immune deficiency states, malnutrition or impaired protein digestion and disturbed metabolism due to liver disease, kidney disease, or anemia.

ALBUMIN/GLOBULIN RATIO

If this level is not in the optimum range it is usually because of changes in the globulin level.

- *Usual:* 0.6 to 2.8
- *Optimum:* 1.4 to 2
- *Mean:* 1.7

CHOLESTEROL

The liver synthesizes most of the cholesterol in the blood; the rest is absorbed from the diet. It is needed for steroid hormone synthesis. A high-saturated fat diet will stimulate the absorption of lipids and cholesterol. If high-density lipoprotein cholesterol is high, the risk of cardiovascular disease is usually lower. Normal values are age dependent.

- *Usual:* 121 to 304 mg/dl
- *Optimum:* 150 to 220 mg/dl
- *Mean:* 212.5 mg/dl

It is elevated in diabetes, liver disease, heart disease, kidney disease, hypothyroidism, hereditary tendency, and pregnancy. High cholesterol is more likely to be associated with low blood pressure. It is lower in malnutrition, hyperthyroidism, liver insufficiency, malignancy, anemia, and infection.

TRIGLYCERIDE

The fat found in the blood after being absorbed from the intestines or converted from glucose and being moved to the fat cells to be stored for future use. A fatty meal will increase this level.

- *Usual:* 30 to 150 mg/dl
- *Optimum:* 50 to 130 mg/dl
- *Mean:* 90 mg/dl

It is elevated if there is poor fat utilization, diabetes, biliary obstruction, kidney disease, alcoholism, liver disease, pancreatitis, hypothyroidism, or use of oral contraceptives. Excess zinc stimulates the conversion of sugars and amino acids to fat.

Low levels are associated with hypoglycemia, stress, malnutrition, or protein metabolism disturbances.

TOTAL BILIRUBIN

This is an indication of the liver's eliminative function. The hemoglobin from dead red blood cells becomes bilirubin and is transported to the liver. It is converted to bile and is passed into the intestines via the bile duct.

- *Usual:* 0.2 to 1.1 mg/dl
- *Optimum:* 0.6 to 0.7 mg/dl
- *Mean:* 0.65 mg/dl

It is elevated in liver disease, bile-duct obstruction, mononucleosis, hemolytic anemia, and toxic effects of drugs (in these situations the whites of the eyes and the skin turn yellow). It is lower if the spleen or liver are inefficient. A diet very low in nitrogen bearing foods might bring the level down.

DIRECT BILIRUBIN

It measures the liver's ability to convert hemoglobin into water-soluble substances so that the kidneys can eliminate them. The test measures the spillover into the circulation.

- *Usual:* 0.0 to 0.3 mg/dl
- *Optimum:* 0.1 to 0.3 mg/dl
- *Mean:* 0.2 mg/dl

It is elevated in liver disease, mononucleosis, or if gall stones are present. It is lowered with severe stress, fatigue, or adrenal gland exhaustion.

ALKALINE PHOSPHATASE

This is an enzyme produced in the cells of the bone or liver. It is most active in an alkaline media. The level rises during degeneration or cell damage, repair, or rapid growth. When the AP is elevated and the liver enzymes are normal, then a bone disease should be considered. It indicates mineral transport into and out of the bone. Injury to bone, pregnancy, or skeletal growth also pushes the level up. Growing children and adolescents have the highest levels.

- *Usual:* 30 to 120 IU/L
- *Optimum:* infancy through adolescence: 50 to 400 IU/L
                     adults: 56 to 105 IU/L
- *Mean:* 75 IU/L

It is elevated in liver disease, mononucleosis, and bone disease. X rays for bone loss should be performed if an adult has a high AP. It is lowered if the adrenal glands are exhausted; there is protein deficiency; malnutrition; magnesium, B_{12}, or vitamin C deficiency; anemia; or hypothyroidism.

LDH

Lactic dehydrogenase is an enzyme in muscles, kidneys, liver, brain, lungs but most abundantly in heart muscle, so an increased amount in the bloodstream indicates damage to one of these tissues. It is at its peak in one to three days after a heart attack. The blood level might reach ten times the normal level. It may even rise with food allergies.

- *Usual:* 100 to 265 IU/L
- *Optimum:* 125 to 240 IU/L
- *Mean:* 182.5 IU/L

Elevations are see in myocardial infarction, leukemia, cancer, anemias, liver disease, embolus in lung, pancreatitis, mononucleosis, or tissue injury. Malnutrition, hypoglycemia, adrenal exhaustion, or a low level of activity of the above-named tissues produce low readings.

GGT

Gamma Glutamyl Transpeptidase is an enzyme found in liver cells.

- *Usual:* males: 5 to 50 IU/L;
            females: 5 to 45 IU/L
- *Optimum:* males: 15 to 45 IU/L;
            females: 10 to 40 IU/L
- *Mean:* males: 27.5 IU/L;
            females: 25 IU/L

It is elevated in bile-duct obstruction, liver disease, alcoholism, and pancreatitis. It might rise with an excessive ingestion of magnesium. It is lowered in hypothyroidism, hypothalamic malfunction, or magnesium deficiency.

SGOT

Serum Glutamic Oxaloacetic Transaminase or ASAT is an enzyme found in cells of the liver, heart, kidney, pancreas, and muscles. If these tissues are damaged—especially the heart and liver—this enzyme level in the blood rises. Its level is used to monitor heart attack progress.

- *Usual:* 6 to 45 IU/L
- *Optimum:* 10 to 40 IU/L
- *Mean:* 25.5 IU/L

It is elevated if a myocardial infarction has occurred (in twenty-four hours after a heart attack it may rise as much as twenty times the upper limits of normal), liver disease, kidney or muscle damage, infection, or mononucleosis. It is lowered in pregnancy and with a vitamin-B deficiency.

SGPT

Serum Glutamic Pyruvic Transaminase or ALAT is an enzyme found mainly in liver cells and less so in heart muscle and other tissues. It spills into the blood with liver damage.

- *Usual:* 0 to 37 IU/L
- *Optimum:* 10 to 35 IU/L
- *Mean:* 18.5 IU/L

It is elevated in liver damage, mononucleosis, alcoholism, kidney infection, chemical pollutants, or myocardial infarction. It is lowered if tissues are not oxygenated properly.

IRON

Iron is required for the production of a number of proteins, namely hemoglobin, myoglobin, and cytochrome. It is necessary for oxygen transport, cellular respiration, and peroxide deactivation. Anemia due to low iron is the most common deficiency disease, especially in menstruating women. It also is necessary for the production of stomach acid.

- *Usual:* 35 to 140 ug/dl
- *Optimum:* 55 to 120 ug/dl

- *Mean:* 87.5 ug/dl

It is elevated in iron overload, hemolytic anemia, liver damage, and pernicious anemia. It is lowered in iron-deficient anemia, deficient bone marrow, senescence, low stomach acid, malabsorption, copper deficiency, zinc excess, low vitamin C, blood loss, liver disease, chronic infections, vegetarian diet, exclusively cow's milk-fed babies, and women with heavy menstrual flow.

TIBC

Total Iron Binding Capacity refers to the available sites for binding of iron in the circulation. If one is low in iron then the capacity for binding will rise.

- *Optimum*: 240 to 400 ug/dl

PERCENT SATURATION

This represents the percentage of the sites saturated with iron. A low percent means there are many sites available; a high percent indicates that most of the sites are occupied.

- *Optimum*: 20 to 55 percent

BLOOD

The transport system, blood carries nutriments out to the cells and brings waste products back to the kidneys, the lungs, and to the liver for detoxification. It brings oxygen and glucose to the cells to supply energy. The blood has red and white cells that account for about 45 percent of the volume. These cells float about in the plasma. When blood clots, the remainder of the blood is called "serum."

Red cells carry the oxygen; the white cells are mainly responsible for fighting infection; and the platelets are needed for clotting.

WBC

The white blood cell count is a measure of the disease-fighting abilities of the blood.

- *Usual range:* 3.8 to 10.5 K/cu mm of blood
- *Optimum range:* 5 to 9 K/cu mm
- *Median:* 7.15 K/cu mm

If the level of the WBC is elevated a bacterial infection is usually taking place. The differential count reveals which group of white cells is elevated. A low level of white cells suggests a weak immune system; a malignant disease is active or the cells are decreased because of some current, overwhelming infection.

RBC

The red blood cell count is responsible for carrying the oxygen to the tissues and the carbon dioxide back to the lungs for exhalation.

- *Usual range:* 3.7 to 5.0 M/cu mm
- *Optimum range:* males: 4.2 to 5.4 M/cu mm
                          females: 4.2 to 4.8 M/cu mm
- *Median:* males: 4.8;
                  females: 4.5 M/cu mm

If the level of the RBCs is up, some toxicity is present; the bone marrow is producing more RBCs because of poor oxygenation or the spleen and liver are not metabolizing properly. The person may be dehydrated. Polycythemia, megaloblastic anemia, B_{12} or folic acid deficiency, bone marrow disease, overingestion of iron are some of the causes of increased RBC. If the level is low, the condition is usually called an anemia, nutritional or genetic. The most common type is iron-poor anemia. Iron, B_{12}, and B_6 are all needed to make RBCs. Poor absorption may be present.

HGB

The hemoglobin is the oxygen carrying protein.

- *Usual range:* 11.2 to 15.2 gm/dl
- *Optimum range:* males: 13.2 to 16.4 gm/dl
                          females: 11.2 to 15.2 gm/dl

- *Mean:* males: 14.8;
     females: 13.2 gm/dl

If the level is abnormally high, some toxin or low oxygen is stimulating the liver to produce more hemoglobin, or excess iron is being ingested, or the liver and spleen are not functioning. A low level of hemoglobin is usually associated with anemia due to lack of iron in the diet, poor nutrition, or a malabsorption problem.

HCT

The hematocrit is a measure of the percentage of the RBCs in whole blood.

- *Usual range:* 35 to 45 percent
- *Optimum range:* males: 40 to 48 percent
                females: 35 to 45 percent
- *Mean:* males: 44
       females: 40

If the level is elevated, it suggests dehydration or a decreased breakdown of RBCs by the spleen. If the level is reduced, it is most likely due to an anemia, or overhydration. An overactive spleen might cause this percent to go down.

MCV

The mean corpuscular volume reflects the size of the red blood cells.

- *Usual range:* 80 to 99 cu mm
- *Optimum:* males: 87 to 94 cu mm
           females: 86 to 92 cu mm

If the level is elevated it means the RBCs are larger than normal (macrocytic anemia). They are usually older cells because the spleen has not destroyed them. If the MCV is reduced, the RBCs are small (microcytic anemia) and oxygen will not get to the tissues efficiently.

MCH

The mean corpuscular hemoglobin gives the average weight of the hemoglobin found in the RBCs.

- *Usual range:* 26 to 34 pico gms
- *Optimum:* 29 to 31 pg

If the level is elevated it means an increase in the amount of hemoglobin in the RBCs, usually due to inadequate oxygenation. If the level is low, the RBCs are pale; it is usually due to lack of iron in the diet.

MCHC

The (mean corpuscular hemoglobin concentration) tells if the average RBC is anemic.

- *Usual range:* 32 to 36 percent
- *Optimum range:* 33 to 35 percent

If the level is elevated, it means hyperchromic anemia. A low level, hypochromic anemia.

THE PLATELET COUNT

These little remnants of cells are always present in the body and help the clotting mechanism.

- *Usual range:* 150 to 450 K/cu mm
- *Optimum range:* 250 to 350 K/cu mm
- *Mean:* 300 K/cu mm

If the level is elevated it suggests dehydration or some stimulation to the bone marrow. If the level is low, the person may bruise more easily. Drugs or an immune system failure may be responsible. Low B_{12} or folic acid may cause a reduction.

THE LYMPHOCYTES

These help to fight infection, produce antibodies, and are sometimes able to control allergies. T-cells are lymphocytes under the control of the thymus gland and help to alert the body to invasion from germs, viruses, and toxins. B-cells are the ones making the antibodies.

- *Optimum level:* 18 to 50 percent of the total white count

If the level is elevated the immune system is active due to some infection. If the count is very low, the immune system is exhausted or the granulocytes are very elevated.

THE MONONUCLEAR CELLS

Help the granulocytes fight infection.

- *Optimum level:* 1 to 9 percent

If the level is elevated, chronic degenerative diseases and tissue breakdown are usually present (tuberculosis, emphysema, or liver infection). A low level is consistent with health.

GRANULOCYTES

The segmented neutrophils help defend the body against infections and antigens.

- *Optimum level:* 42 to 75 percent of the total count

If the level is elevated, an acute infection is in progress. The immune system is being challenged.

BANDS

The bands are immature granulocytes or polymorphonuclear neutrophils.

- *Optimum:* less than 3 percent of the differential count

They are elevated if an infection was active at the time of the blood withdrawal. If under 3 percent, no infection is active.

MONOCYTES

The monocytes are usually considered part of the mononuclear group of cells and have the same significance.

EOSINOPHILS

Named thusly because they stain red with a dye called eosin, the eosinophils help protect against allergic reactions and parasites.

- *Optimum*: less than 4 percent of the total white count

If elevated, an allergy is in progress. Parasites will raise the eosinophil count. A low level is compatible with health.

BASOPHILS

They carry histamine, which is responsible for some allergic reactions.

- *Optimum*: less than 2 percent of the total white count

They are elevated with drug reactions, some parasitic infections, and some allergies. A low count is normal.

ANION/CATION

This is the figure resulting from the subtraction of the acidic factors in the blood from the alkaline factors. It is figured by this method (sodium + potassium) − (CO_2 + chloride) = measure of acidity or alkalinity. (See next chapter.)

- *Values of 6 to 12* are considered normal
- *Values of below 6* are considered in the acid range
- *Values of above 12* are considered in the alkaline range
(that person will feel better on the acidifiers: ammonium chloride, betaine hydrochloride, and/or vinegar).

If most of your blood tests are within the range the laboratory considers normal, your doctor will reassure you that "Your tests all seem to be normal. The exam I performed shows that you are fairly healthy for a person of your age. Your aches, pains, and fatigue are a part of growing old.''

Before he/she suggests a prescription for a sleeping pill, a tranquilizer, a muscle relaxant, or atonic, you should ask for a copy of the blood test, saying, ''For my own records.''

When you get home, you can sort out the values depending on their value above or below the mean. The Life Balances program has a computer method that accurately divides up the results into too much or too little, and can do it in a twinkling. The next chapter contains the printout from the computer that has sorted out the data.

11

How to Read
and Interpret
the Blood Tests

The resulting printout obtained from the computer analysis of the laboratory results is the heart of the Life Balances program. It tells several things about the person's physiology on the day the blood was drawn. With this data and the completed questionnaire before him, Mr. Kitkoski determines what supplements the client should take to become healthy and energetic. He feels that although people should take more responsibility for their own health, they should be working in cooperation with a health care professional who would be able to monitor the progress.

Note: No one who follows the advice in this book should stop their prescribed medicines in the hope that Life Balances will solve their disease problems overnight.

But can you do something yourself with this information? We all get sick. We all get old. We all have aches and pains. We have mood swings. We get depressed. We want to maintain an ideal weight for our body type. We have embarrassing cravings and addictions. We have a hard time making our bodies do exactly what we want. So take a little responsibility for your health. It's all quite safe if you follow the smelling and tasting rules.

Here are a few chemical truisms the readers can note for themselves. The suggestions are safe to try.

Positive and Negative Values

Compare the positive values (values greater than the mean) with the negative values (values less than the mean) in the column on the right side of the printout. If there are more negative values than positive values, the subject is nutrient-deficient, like balsa wood, and needs supplements, especially the minerals. The deviation figure at the bottom of the right-hand column will have a negative value less than − 2 percent. (The laboratory we use has recently made a few changes in the ranges—see the columns "High" and "Low" on Table 11.1—due to more information. These adjustments have only marginal effects on the final readings.)

Not enough of the building blocks are present to make the enzymes necessary for optimal functioning. The subject may have been unable or unwilling to eat enough food containing the proteins, the carbohydrates, and the varieties of minerals required by busy organs and tissues. If people are nutrient-deficient, they usually are tired with cold hands and feet. Many are depressed and sickly. A poor immune system is often associated with negative deviations below the mean. Simultaneous with his improved health and energy, the negative values on the blood test rise and cluster closer to the mean. The allergies become less bothersome. Even hypochondriacs complain less. The mineral drops are often useful for this participant.

If the percent deviation is greater than + 2, the client is nutrient-dense; the higher the percent, the higher the density, like teak wood. In this case extra water and the electrolytes are needed to move water into the tissues and make the vitamins and minerals more soluble.

The person whose blood is analyzed in the next three pages (see Tables 11.1 and 11.2) is nutrient dense (deviation at the bottom is 5.1%), mildly alkaline (Anion/Cation at 11.2 is at the upper end of normal), and has been taking too much magnesium (as shown by the elevated GGT). At time went by, his hands and feet warmed up and his calcium came up close to the mean because daily he had been drinking 2% milk mixed half and half with the electrolyte solution. But from August, 1989, to April, 1990, he slacked off on the milk and electrolyte; his calcium level dropped off. These three pages show how the computer can reveal if a person is or is not following the rules. This person has a way to go yet.

Anion/Cation Ratio

The anion/cation ratio indicates the degree of acidity or alkalinity present at the time of the blood-draw. Most people in North

TABLE 11.1
BLOOD TEST EVALUATION

Results		Low	High	Mean	+ or − Mean	Weighted Deviation from Mean
GGT	103.0	0.0	55.0	27.5	75.5	137.27%
Total Bilirubin	1.2	0.2	1.1	0.65	0.6	61.11%
Triglycerides	143.0	30.0	150.0	90.0	53.0	44.17%
Anion/Cation	11.2	6.0	12.0	9.0	2.2	36.67%
Hemoglobin	15.9	13.2	16.4	14.8	1.1	34.38%
MCHC	35.3	32.0	36.0	34.0	1.3	33.33%
Neutrophils	66.0	42.0	75.0	58.5	7.5	22.73%
MCH	31.8	26.0	34.0	30.0	1.8	22.50%
Chloride	105.0	95.0	109.0	102.0	3.0	21.43%
Cholesterol	250.0	121.0	304.0	212.5	37.5	20.49%
RBC	5.0	4.2	5.4	4.8	0.2	16.67%
Uric Acid	6.2	3.7	7.6	5.65	0.6	14.10%
Hematocrit	45.0	40.0	48.0	44.0	1.0	12.50%
Glucose-Fasting	93.0	65.0	110.0	87.5	5.5	12.22%
Platelet Est.	325.0	140.0	440.0	290.0	35.0	11.67%
Albumin	4.4	3.5	5.0	4.25	0.2	10.00%
BUN	17.0	8.0	23.0	15.5	1.5	10.00%
CO_2	28.0	23.0	32.0	27.5	0.5	5.56%
Sodium/Potassium	33.33	26.91	38.6	32.76	0.6	4.90%
WBC	7.4	3.8	10.5	7.15	0.3	3.73%
Iron	111.0	55.0	160.0	107.5	3.5	3.33%
Total Protein	6.9	6.0	7.7	6.85	0.1	2.94%
A/G Ratio	1.8	0.6	2.8	1.7	0.1	2.73%
MCV	90.0	80.0	99.0	89.5	0.5	2.63%
SGOT	23.0	5.0	40.0	22.5	0.5	1.43%
SGPT	19.0	0.0	37.0	18.5	0.5	1.35%
Creatinine	1.1	0.8	1.4	1.1	0.0	0.00%
Sodium	140.0	135.0	145.0	140.0	0.0	0.00%
Basophils	1.0	0.0	2.0	1.0	0.0	0.00%
Chloride/CO_2	3.75	3.2	4.4	3.8	− 0.1	− 4.17%
Potassium	4.2	3.4	5.2	4.3	− 0.1	− 5.56%
Alk. Phosphatase	68.0	30.0	120.0	75.0	− 7.0	− 7.78%
LDH	153.0	90.0	240.0	165.0	− 12.0	− 8.00%
Phosphorus	3.3	2.5	4.5	3.5	− 0.2	− 10.00%
BUN/Creat Ratio	15.5	6.0	30.0	18.0	− 2.5	− 10.61%
Globulin	2.5	1.6	4.0	2.8	− 0.3	− 12.50%
Lymphocytes	28.0	15.0	50.0	32.5	− 4.5	− 12.86%
Monocytes	4.0	1.0	10.0	5.5	− 1.5	− 16.67%
Eosinophils	1.0	0.0	4.0	2.0	− 1.0	− 25.00%
Calcium	8.8	8.5	10.5	9.5	− 0.7	− 35.00%
Ionized Ca	3.9	3.8	4.8	4.3	− 0.4	− 38.51%
Ca/P Ratio	2.67	2.6	3.2	2.9	− 0.2	− 38.89%
Bands	0.0	0.0	5.0	2.5	− 2.5	− 50.00%
Atyp. Lymphocyte	0.0	0.0	7.0	3.5	− 3.5	− 50.00%

AVG. DEVIATION   19.89%
+ OR − DEVIATION   5.10%

Electrolytes	Weighted Deviation from the Mean
Sodium	0.00%
Potassium	−5.56%
Chloride	21.43%
CO$_2$	5.56%
Calcium	−35.00%
Total Deviation	13.51%
+ or − Deviation	−2.71%

Renal Function	Weighted Deviation from the Mean
BUN	10.00%
Chloride	21.43%
CO$_2$	5.56%
Creatinine	0.00%
Potassium	−5.56%
Sodium	0.00%
Total Deviation	7.09%
+ or − Deviation	5.24%

Liver	Weighted Deviation from the Mean
SGOT	1.43%
SGPT	1.35%
GGT	137.27%
T. Bilirubin	61.11%
Alk. Phosphatase	−7.78%
Total Deviation	41.79%
+ or − Deviation	38.68%

Lipids	Weighted Deviation from the Mean
Cholesterol	20.49%
Triglycerides	44.17%
Total Deviation	32.33%
+ or − Deviation	32.33%

Hematology	Weighted Deviation from the Mean
WBC	3.73%
RBC	16.67%
Hemoglobin	34.38%
Hematocrit	12.50%
MCV	2.63%
MCH	22.50%
MCHC	33.33%
Platelets	11.67%
Total Deviation	17.18%
+ or − Deviation	17.18%

Differential WBC	Weighted Deviation from the Mean
Neutrophils	22.73%
Bands	−50.00%
Lymphocytes	−12.86%
Monocytes	−16.67%
Eosinophils	−25.00%
Basophils	0.00%
Atyp. Lymphs	−50.00%
Total Deviation	25.32%
+ or − Deviation	−18.83%

Ratios	Weighted Deviation from the Mean
Anion/Cation	36.67%
Ca/P	−38.89%
Na/K	4.90%
Cl/CO$_2$	−4.17%
BUN/Creat	−10.61%
Total Deviation	19.05%
+ or − Deviation	−2.42%

Proteins	Weighted Deviation from the Mean
T. Protein	2.94%
Albumin	10.00%
Globulin	−12.50%
A/G Ratio	2.73%
Total Deviation	7.04%
+ or − Deviation	0.79%

TABLE 11.2
BLOOD TEST COMPARISON

	First Test (8/18/89)	Second Test (4/11/90)	First Test: Dev. from Mean	Second Test: Dev. from Mean	Change
Total Bilirubin	1.5	1.2	94.44%	61.11%	33.33%
Sodium/Potassum	29.58	33.33	−35.63%	−3.91%	31.72%
Chloride/CO$_2$	4.00	3.75	31.99%	−2.53%	29.46%
MCV	96	90	31.85%	2.63%	29.21%
Total Protein	6.4	6.9	−26.47%	2.94%	23.53%
Potassium	4.8	4.2	27.78%	−5.56%	22.22%
Chloride	108	105	42.86%	21.43%	21.43%
Globulin	2.0	2.5	−33.33%	−12.50%	20.83%
Phosphorus	2.9	3.3	−30.00%	−10.00%	20.00%
Sodium	142	140	20.00%	0.00%	20.00%
A/G Ratio	2.2	1.8	22.73%	2.73%	20.00%
Iron	84	111	−22.38%	3.33%	19.05%
Uric Acid	6.8	6.2	29.49%	14.10%	15.38%
WBC	5.9	7.4	−18.66%	3.73%	14.93%
Ca/P Ratio	3.21	2.67	51.15%	−38.89%	12.26%
Alk Phosphatase	57	68	−20.00%	−7.78%	12.22%
LDH	137	153	−18.67%	−8.00%	10.67%
Anion/Cation	11.8	11.2	46.67%	36.67%	10.00%
MCH	32.4	31.8	30.19%	22.50%	7.69%
Glucose-Fasting	96	93	18.89%	12.22%	6.67%
SGPT	16	19	−6.76%	1.35%	5.41%
BUN/Creat Ratio	14.5	15.5	−14.39%	−10.61%	3.79%
Hematocrit	45.1	45	13.75%	12.50%	1.25%
Lymphocytes	27.8	28	−13.43%	−12.86%	0.57%
Neutrophils	66.1	66	23.03%	22.73%	0.30%
Creatinine	1.1	1.1	0.00%	0.00%	0.00%
Triglycerides	143	143	44.17%	44.17%	0.00%
Albumin	4.4	4.4	10.00%	10.00%	0.00%
SGOT	22	23	−1.43%	1.43%	0.00%
CO$_2$	27	28	−5.56%	5.56%	0.00%
Bands	0	0	−50.00%	−50.00%	0.00%
Eosinophils	1	1	−25.00%	−25.00%	0.00%
Basophils	1	1	0.00%	0.00%	0.00%
BUN	16	17	3.33%	10.00%	−6.67%
Platelet Est.	296	325	−1.33%	8.33%	−7.00%
Monocytes	6.1	4	6.67%	−16.67%	−10.00%
RBC	4.72	5	−6.67%	16.67%	−10.00%
Cholesterol	229	250	9.02%	20.49%	−11.48%
Hemoglobin	15.3	15.9	15.63%	34.38%	−18.75%
Calcium	9.3	8.8	−10.00%	−35.00%	−25.00%
MCHC	33.9	35.3	−1.88%	33.33%	−31.45%
Ionized Calcium	4.3	3.9	2.81%	−38.51%	−35.70%
GGT	82	103	99.09%	137.27%	−38.18%

AVERAGE PERCENT DEVIATION   24.15%   18.59%

AVERAGE + OR − DEVIATION   7.88%   7.20%

America are in some alkalosis, i.e., the value is above 12. Here is a sample, and rather a typical situation:

(sodium at 140 + potassium at 4.3) − (CO_2 at 27.5 + chloride at 102)
144.3 minus 129.5
equals
14.8

This is moderate alkalosis as the value is above 12. It appears that even if a person is "perfect" because his values are right on the mean, he can still be alkaline. The explanation seems to be that the labs have found most of the tests of people living in North America average out as being in the alkaline range. Being right on the mean or perfectly average in North America pushes one into alkalinity. Our diet and our lifestyle determine this. We see many with a score close to 20, and most of them have muscle aches and spasms. One little boy with seizures had a score of 25! Drugs to control the spells put him to sleep. His sodium was very high. When he drank a *pint* of vinegar a day, he was almost seizure free, but at least needed fewer drugs.

Alkalosis is usually associated with allergies, asthma, muscle aches and spasms, migraines, spastic colon, insomnia, bed-wetting, and even bad breath. Most people who have this elevated anion/cation ratio can be helped with either vinegar if the sodium is up and their blood pressure is elevated, or the ammonium chloride if they are not.

If a person has been alkaline since childhood, he usually has crowded lower front teeth. It difficult for the minerals to be effective in alkalosis during the metabolic processes because minerals must be in an acidic medium to be soluble. The minerals, therefore, are not available to allow for the normal development of the jaw. Calcium, magnesium, and iron require acidification to be usable. Ammonium chloride (NH_4Cl) is usually necessary to reduce alkalosis and promote acidity. Betaine HCl is useful for acidification also.

Nitrogen-bearing Compounds

If the uric acid, the BUN, and the creatinine are low, it suggests that nitrogen is not getting into the body or being utilized properly. Ammonium chloride may be helpful in providing more nitrogen.

Amino acids and a high-protein diet are necessary for a few weeks. Hormones are built on nitrogen. BUN should be higher than the uric acid. Bilirubin is high or low depending upon the intestinal flora. The nitrogen cycle is important to teeth and bones.

Calcium

Check the calcium level. Calcium regulates the osmolarity of the tissues and regulates the sodium/potassium ratio (Na/K). Large-boned people are high in calcium and have large veins. Calcium and phosphate are needed for growth. Frequent salad eaters get a fair amount of calcium and eventually might develop high blood pressure. Broccoli yields calcium and potassium, both alkaline foods. Calcium makes nitrogen available for use. Calcium thins the blood. Low calcium is associated with hypothermia.

Sodium

Sodium tightens the muscles. Sodium is high if the biceps are large; sodium affects the front muscles. Men are usually high in sodium. Sodium is needed to carry the calcium to the bones. Low sodium, acidic people have low blood pressure in the A.M. and higher in the P.M. High-sodium, alkaline people have high blood pressure in the A.M. with lower blood pressure in the P.M., as some calcium and the sodium leave the tissues during the night. Sodium affects the blood pressure from 90 mm mercury and higher. If the sodium is elevated and the systolic pressure is up, vinegar will reduce the pressure, especially if the client is overweight. If the sodium and the blood pressure are low, that person will dislike vinegar. Sodium bicarbonate ($NaHCO_3$) ingestion leads to high blood pressure.

If a person has flexion-type seizures (body bends forward, arms and legs flex on to the trunk), he is usually high in sodium and low in potassium.

Potassium

Potassium (K) levels drop during emotional stresses; "died of a broken heart." An electrolyte high in potassium stabilizes emotions. Potassium affects the backside muscles. If a person has seizures and arches backward with his limbs extended, it means he has an excess of potassium and a lack of sodium. Potassium builds the triceps (back muscles of upper arms). Potassium loosens muscles. Women have higher potassium levels than men. Potassium affects the blood pressure from 90 mm of mercury and below.

Magnesium

The relative amount of magnesium can be inferred by the amount of GGT. This enzyme is magnesium-dependent; when little magnesium is present, the GGT is lower than average. Magnesium helps control allergies.

The exciting part of the program to most people is the close correlation between the sensory selection of the supplements and the blood values. This serves to illustrate the science, the uniqueness, and the reliability of this methodology. A daily blood test is not necessary to determine one's daily requirements. The blood tests give the general guidelines for the direction that must be taken, and then the daily evaluation of supplement needs can rest on the senses. Smell and taste will allow daily control to be specific because bodily needs will change each day depending upon the diet and the omnipresent stressors. The daily monitoring provides the fine control.

After you, the amateur chemist, diagnostician, therapist has looked over your blood tests and noted that you are (1) above the mean in your sodium level, (2) below the mean in your calcium and (3) GGT, you now should check the correlation between symptoms and signs as listed in Chapter 6.

Now for (1) above, try a teaspoon of apple cider vinegar in an eight-ounce glass of water. If your sodium is above the mean, this will taste good to you. You may drink that mixture two to three times a day as long as it tastes good to you. Your systolic blood pressure will fall if its elevation was due to a high sodium level in your blood.

For (2) above, smell a bottle of calcium (Life Balances is the best source because of purity). It should smell good or have no smell. You need it just as the calcium-below-the mean test indicates. Drinking cow's milk modified for absorption with the electrolyte (1/2 and 1/2) is a satisfactory way to get calcium and some other nutrients into the system.

For (3) above, smell a bottle of magnesium from L.B. It should smell good or have no smell. You need it. (See symptoms of magnesium deficiency in Chapter 6, pages 51–52.)

You are on your way.

12

Choosing the Life Balances Therapy

So now you have dipped into the program; it is making sense to you. You are getting the "AHA!" feeling. But, "will my doctor understand if I want to try the LB program? Will he/she pout or get mad and throw me out because I am challenging his/her therapy?" I have a urologist who wants to ream out my prostate because it is enlarged, and he was trained to do that surgery, and he does it well. However, saw palmetto and L.B. control my nocturia. My wife tends to have high blood pressure and her doctor wants her on a diuretic. However, when she conscientiously and consistently follows the L.B. program, her blood pressure is reasonably normal. She hates drugs.

You will find doctors who are interested in this program, and who can direct and guide you through the steps to attain a chemical, metabolic balance. Everything this book has told you is compatible with whatever your primary physician wants you to do. This program runs parallel to using prescription drugs, having a chiropractor adjust you, working with a naturopathic physician, or allowing a medical doctor do a history and physical exam and coming up with a prescription.

Following is a list of fairly common diseases and conditions and the various modalities of care that are available. You can choose your favorite method of control or combination of treatments. Life Balances works along with the treatments outlined, and may, in some cases, be the only therapy needed. You can try Life Balances without your doctor's knowledge. Then when he/she notices that you are better, he will (1) ask what you have been doing or (2) know it was his/her therapy that fixed you. Either way, you win.

We have found that many herbal remedies, helpful though they may be, are somewhat alkaline, and might interfere with any acidification attempt. In any event, much like any form of treatment, the size of the dosage is important. Too little can be useless; too much can be dangerous. Talk to your herbalist or naturopathic physician.

Some Disease Control Choices

ACNE

Allopathic control: Cleanse the skin, broad-spectrum antibiotics to control infections Retin-A (vitamin A analog). Does not address the reason for the acne. The antibiotics usually cause an increase in the yeast, *Candida*.

Natural control: Change to a high-fiber diet; no milk, cola, chocolate, nuts, or sugar. Use only small amounts of iodine or fat.

Increase intake of vitamins A and C, pantothenic acid, zinc, B$_6$, and essential fatty acids. Apply to skin: Comfrey gel and *Calendula*. Herbs: burdock root, dandelion root, *Echinacea*, kelp, alfalfa, chaparral, yellow dock root, red clover, lymph, *Natrum muriaticum*, *Kalium bromatum*, *Juglans nigra*, *Ledum palustre*, *Hepar sulphuris*, *Calcareum*, garlic, fenugreek, red sage, *Lactobacillus acidophilus*.

ADENOIDS

Allopathic control: Surgical removal, usually including the tonsils.

Natural control: Diet change, especially avoid milk. If infected, five grams of vitamin C plus *Echinacea*—ten days on, then ten days off. Other useful herbs: *Hydrastis*, *Berberis*.

AGING

Allopathic control: Nursing home, periodic checks for cancer, blood pressure.

Natural control: Exercise and a low-fat diet with supplements, particularly vitamins C, A and E. Herbal treatments: *Angelica*, *Ginkgo biloba*, Siberian ginseng, Panax ginseng, dandelion, gentian, horehound, licorice, *Cassia*, parsley, saw palmetto.

ALCOHOLISM

Allopathic control: Alcoholics Anonymous, tranquilizers.

Natural control: Change diet—eat every two to three hours—extra protein, add vitamins A, C and B-complex, calcium, magnesium, zinc, and L-glutamine. No sugar. Rule out food sensitivities and hypoglycemia. Acupuncture. Herbal remedies: *Lactobacillus acidophilus*, *Nux vomica*, *Avena sativa*.

ALOPECIA

Allopathic control: Local injections of cortisone.

Natural control: Avoid stress, and cleanse the liver with a new diet. No sugar.

Life Balances program: The chem screen shows generalized nutritional problems and deficiencies—they need: protein and correction of alkalinity, as well as multiple minerals and vitamins.

Alopecia

Here follows the brief story of two women who have suffered from alopecia totalis.

CASE #1: L.A.B.

L.A.B. began the program in January 1990. Female, forty-four years, 122 pounds, 5 feet, 8 inches. Advertising business. Divorced. College and post-graduate education.

At age twenty-three she began to have patchy baldness. By 1986 (age forty) had alopecia totalis (scalp, armpits, pubic—total). She feels that stress two to three months before the loss began was a trigger to the problem. She tried diet, cortisone, acupuncture, vitamins, ginseng, castor oil packs, visualization, and massage—all to no avail. Had asthma and backaches also, but they are less severe now. Some hay fever. Uterine fibroids caused stomachaches. Not a smoker. One glass of wine with dinner. Occasional use of aspirin. Had one abortion. Occasional mucus in throat, occasional coughing, some gas, bloat, and heartburn. Occasional attack of herpes, both genital and oral. Occasional

(continued on page 126)

(continued from page 125)

headaches, especially before her menses. She stopped dairy products because of *Candida*. She avoids meat. AIDS test negative. BP 120/80.

The alopecia was patchy for ten years. After age thirty-seven it got worse and by age thirty-eight all her hair was gone. Also had bad backaches when all her hair fell out.

She has not followed the program carefully or consistently. Some hair started to grow in during the fall of 1990, but now in 1993, it is just a light fuzz. Backaches are still present.

L.A.B.	Jan 1990	Mar 1990	July 1990	Oct 1990	Feb 1991	Nov 1991
Ani/Cation	+105%	+121%	+93%	+40%	+73%	+42%
Chloride	+28%	+36%	0%	+18%	+18%	+13%
Protein	+14%	+3%	−14%	−2%	−30%	+2%
Uric acid	−9%	−25%	−56%	−46%	−58%	−48%
GGT	−16%	−20%	−19%	−26%	−33%	−19%
Cholesterol	−19%	−24%	−27%	−19%	−22%	−22%
Calcium	−20%	+5%	+7%	+7%	−21%	−2%
BUN	−23%	−30%	−22%	−33%	−44%	−28%
Triglyceride	−28%	+10%	−35%	−31%	−31%	−25%
Ion calcium	−31%	−1%	+3%	−7%	−10%	−9%
CO_2	−50%	−50%	0%	−7%	−14%	−7%
avg % dev	+27%	+28%	+22%	+28%	+27%	+19%
% + or − deviation	+3%	+2%	−4%	+8%	−5%	−3%

These plus or minus percent deviations from the mean indicate that L.A.B. was unable to follow the directions of the program. She became less alkaline over the 22 months that she stayed with the program, but she did not eat enough protein as seen by the low levels of BUN, Uric acid and cholesterol and triglycerides. This may explain why she has been only able to grow a little fuzz. The low levels of GGT (indicate low magnesium) shows that she is still under some stress and anxiety. The lab test also showed she was low in sodium and should have taken in more salt.

(continued on page 127)

(continued from page 126)

The average percent deviation should have approached a more normal value of less than 20% after the first few months. The % + or − should be in the + 2% to − 2% range if she had become balanced.

CASE #2: K.R.

K.R., female, age forty-three years, about 130 pounds, 5 feet, 3 inches. Hysterectomy age thirty-three. Placed on Estrace. In January 1988, age thirty-eight, went through a traumatic divorce. Began to notice patches of baldness in September 1989: Alopecia areata. Visited many dermatologists: Anthraline, cortisone injections of no benefit. Hormones from OB/Gyn of no benefit. Endocrinologist found underactive thyroid in spring 1990, and prescribed Synthroid. Hair continued to fall out. Wanted to try vitamins, but did not know which or how much.

K.R.	Sept 1990	Jan 1991	Apr 1991	Aug 1991	Feb 1992	July 1992	Jan 1993
Ani/Cation	+ 48%	+ 147%	+ 83%	+ 50%	+ 50%	+ 80%	+ 85%
Chloride	+ 30%	+ 6%	+ 12%	− 6%	0%	+ 30%	+ 23%
CO_2	+ 25%	− 29%	0%	+ 21%	− 7%	− 21%	0%
BUN	+ 7%	− 17%	− 22%	− 22%	− 5%	− 17%	− 11%
Albumin	+ 3%	− 7%	− 7%	− 7%	− 2%	− 15%	+ 2%
Iron	− 2%	+ 38%	+ 2%	+ 10%	+ 7%	+ 39%	+ 6%
Cholsterol	− 6%	− 16%	− 22%	− 13%	− 11%	− 18%	− 23%
GGT	− 8%	− 24%	− 30%	− 17%	+ 10%	+ 17%	+ 21%
Sodium	− 10%	− 4%	+ 4%	− 12%	− 35%	− 12%	+ 4%
Calcium	− 17%	− 7%	− 11%	− 12%	− 21%	− 21%	+ 2%
Triglycrds	− 20%	+ 10%	− 8%	− 13%	− 15%	+ 10%	− 17%
Uric Acid	− 27%	− 60%	− 28%	− 26%	− 36%	− 46%	− 38%
Potassium	− 29%	+ 22%	+ 33%	+ 33%	+ 33%	+ 22%	+ 38%
Ion Ca	− 35%	− 17%	− 15%	− 12%	− 38%	− 25%	− 15%
avg % dev	18%	21%	25%	18%	21%	19%	17%
% + or − deviation	3%	− 3%	− 2.7	− 5%	− 2%	− 2%	− 1%

(continued on page 128)

(continued from page 127)

Started Life Balances in November 1990. Had trouble because the vitamins and minerals made her nauseated and fatigued. She was exhausted, pale, and her nails were ridged and pitted. Had to take a leave of absence from work. By January 1991, she had not one hair on head or body. Even nasal hairs were gone. Very depressed. Alopecia totalis universalis. In spring of 1991, her stamina improved. Back to work in April. May 1991 a few hairs started on scalp but they fell out soon afterward. Cold sores continued, but her color and stamina improved. In September 1991, fuzz appeared on face and crown of head. Her total protein improved from a − 18 percent to a + 2 percent in February 1992. "I was actually synthesizing hair. This was my turning point." July 1992: Pores changing. Body fuzz in patches on neck and one blond eyelash showed up. Nails are almost normal. "It has been a slow but steady story of progress. Every day I have more and more hair. My energy level seems on a par with my peers. Sometimes even stronger. Mostly I feel normal in the flow of life, instead of trying to run alongside desperately trying to keep up. Life is for the healthy." Keep people healthy is better than "coming in the back door of sickness with treatments." "What money could be saved.?! What life could be saved!?"

AMENORRHEA

Allopathic control: Rule out diseases and confirm or deny pregnancy, hormone therapy with estrogen and progesterone (synthetic).

Natural control: Avoid exercise and stress, use nourishing diet. Herbs: Black cohosh, *Vitex, Angelica.*

ANEMIA

Allopathic control: B_{12} for pernicious, iron for hypochromic anemia, find reason for blood loss.

Natural control: Find food sensitivities; stop drinking milk. Use whole foods, B_{12}, iron fumarate, may need all the B-complex vitamins, A, C, E, copper, zinc. Check for low stomach acid. Herbal remedies: Nettles, red clover, yellow dock, burdock.

ANOREXIA NERVOSA

Allopathic control: Hospitalization and psychiatric treatment.

Natural control: Eliminate stress, add zinc and essential fatty acids. Herbs: Chamomile, gentian root, ginger.

ARTHRITIS

Allopathic control: Aspirin, nonsteroidal antiinflammatory drugs (usually have side effects).

Natural control: Chinese herbs, VEGA testing for food allergies, stool exam for ova and parasites. Vitamins and nutrients: B_6, copper, vegan diet, pantothenic acid, C, manganese, selenium, sulfur, zinc, essential fatty acids. Herbs: Alfalfa, yucca root, celery seed, burdock root, sarsaparilla root, *Capsicum*, queen of the meadows, devil's claw.

Life Balances program: Check blood for alkalinity and nutrient deficiencies. (People with osteoarthritis are more comfortable in Florida because of the high humidity and higher phosphates in their diet. Those with rheumatoid arthritis are more likely to enjoy Arizona because of the low humidity and the increased amounts of nitrogen in the air.)

BACKACHE

Allopathic control: Nonsteroidal antiinflammatories.

Natural control: Massage, adjustments, and exercises. Increase use of calcium, magnesium, potassium, and vitamin E. Herbal remedies: Alfalfa, yucca root, celery seed, burdock root, *Capsicum*, *Valerian*.

BAD BREATH (Halitosis)

Allopathic control: Control gum disease and bad teeth; control postnasal drip; use mouthwash; and stop eating garlic and onions.

Natural control: If above do not work, change diet, cleanse bowels. Increase intake of Chlorophyll and *Lactobacillus acidophilus*. Herbal cures: Dandelion root, yellow dock, *Capsicum*, burdock, red clover, mint, anise, fennel.

BONE SPURS

Allopathic control: Surgical removal.

Natural control: Ultrasound, massage.

BREAST CYSTS

Allopathic control: Surgery. X ray to rule out cancer.

Natural control: Stop drinking caffeine, coffee, and soft drinks. Add vitamins B_6, A, E, iodine, omega-6 fatty acids. Other dietary supplements: Licorice, *Lactobacillus acidophilus*.

BREAST FEEDING

Allopathic control: Refer to lactation expert; drink two quarts of milk a day.

Natural control: Rotate the diet and take supplements. Herbs: Fenugreek, fennel, anise, borage, goat's rue.

BURSITIS

Allopathic control: Injection with steroids.

Natural control: Deep heat, ultrasound, B_{12} injections, plus vitamin C, and bioflavonoids.

CARDIAC ARRHYTHMIA

Allopathic control: Digitalis, calcium channel blockers, other drugs, pacemaker.

Natural control: Avoid caffeine and stimulants; no aspartame or cayenne pepper. Excessive zinc and deficient copper may cause this. Magnesium may help, as may: calcium, potassium, carnitine, coenzyme Q_{10}, taurine, C, E, B-complex, garlic, lecithin, kelp, and essential fatty acids. Herbs: hawthorne berries, valerian root, dandelion, barberry, red grape vine leaves, *Crataegus oxyacantha*, valeriana, *Kalium phosphoricum*, *Amni visnaga*.

CARPAL TUNNEL SYNDROME

Allopathic control: Splints. Surgery.

Natural control: Splints, B_6.

CATARACT

Allopathic control: Surgery and lens replacement

Natural control: Change diet: no sugar; add riboflavin, C, E, cod liver oil, selenium, zinc, and cysteine.

CELIAC DISEASE

Allopathic control: No glutens.

Natural control: No glutens; add folic acid, B_{12}, B_6, A, D, E, K, iron, and selenium. Herbs: *Aloe vera*, gentian, slippery elm, marshmallow root.

CHOLESTEROL

Allopathic control: Stop eggs, butter, use skim milk, prescribe niacin and cholesteramine.

Natural control: vegetarian diet, use skim milk, cut sugar from diet. Other dietary supplements: *Lactobacillus acidophilus* and *Cammaphora gugul.*

CIRRHOSIS OF LIVER

Allopathic control: Stop drinking, join AA.

Natural control: Sylibum, low-fat diet, extra vitamins, especially the Bs. Herbs: *Tang kuei*, *Carthamus*, *Spiriferis tossila*, *Taraxacum*, artichoke leaves, curamin.

COLD HANDS AND FEET

Allopathic control: Massage, hot water bottle, wear socks to bed.

Natural control: Check thyroid; improve circulation with herbs; and drink water. Herbs: *Capsicum*, *Crataegus*, *Ginkgo*, linsen flower.

COLIC

Allopathic control: Drugs; change formula.

Natural control: Chamomile tea, fennel seed, anise, change diet. If breast-fed, change mother's diet.

COLITIS

Allopathic control: Add roughage, tranquilizers.

Natural control: Vega testing of parotid secretin, pancreas secretin, stomach secretin, small and large intestine secretin, liver secretin, gallbladder secretin for sensitivities to: milk, wheat, eggs, corn, and soy.

CONSTIPATION

Allopathic control: Add roughage, bulk laxatives.

Natural control: Change diet: stop dairy, white flour, and sugar; add roughage and *Psyllium* seeds.

CROHN'S DISEASE

Allopathic control: Prednisone, asulfidine, bland diet.

*Natural control:*Hypoallergenic diet: no sugar; add folic acid, B-complex, C, A, B_{12}, D, K, calcium, magnesium, selenium, and zinc.

CYSTIC FIBROSIS

Allopathic control: Vitamin A, postural drainage, antibiotics, pancreatic enzymes.

Natural control: Vitamins A, C, E, Herbs: *Echinacea, Gundelia,* mullein.

DANDRUFF

Allopathic control: Special shampoos; salicylate ointments.

Natural control: Take vitamins A and E, pyridoxine, zinc, primrose oil, lecithin, and kelp; use calendula cream. No fatty foods, dairy, sugar, or chocolate. Herbs: Red clover, dandelion, golden seal.

DIABETES

Allopathic control: Insulin; balanced diet; three meals a day; a snack at bedtime.

Natural control: Search for food sensitivities. Change to a high-fiber diet; no sugar; add zinc, chromium, brewer's yeast, biotin, B_6, copper, manganese, and magnesium. Herbs: *Lycopodium, Pancreatinum, Gymnea,* devil's club, *Taraxacum,* blueberry leaf, jambul.

DIARRHEA

Allopathic control: Fast, intravenous fluids with electrolytes; stool culture.

Natural control: Eat bananas, rice, applesauce, and toast. Supplement diet with: Agrimony, blackberry root, *Rhus toxicodendron, Phosphoricum acidum, Ferrum phosphoricum. Lactobacillus acidophilus.*

DIVERTICULOSIS (and Diverticulitis)

Allopathic control: Add roughage; surgery if painful.

Natural control: Food allergy tests. Add fiber, vitamins A, B-complex and C; aloe-vera juice; acidophilus; proteolytic enzymes; multidigestive enzymes; magnesium; zinc; and chromium.

DYSPEPSIA

Allopathic control: Antacids, Valium.

Natural control: Take digestive enzymes with meals; order a Vega test for food sensitivities; and increase intake of fiber, B-complex, raw duodenal concentrate, pepsin, lipotrophic factors, and kyolic garlic. Herbs: Aloe-vera juice, acidophilus, chamomile, fennel, catnip, slippery elm, marshmallow root, pepsin, gentian root.

DYSMENORRHEA

Allopathic control: Aspirin; codeine; exercise; synthetic hormones; hysterectomy.

Natural control: Add niacin, B_6, magnesium, E, iron (if anemic), and essential fatty acids to diet.

EDEMA

Allopathic control: Check for heart, liver, or kidney failure. Use diuretics.

Natural control: If above diseases are ruled out, use B_6, vitamins C and E, calcium, magnesium, alfalfa, and silicon. Increase raw foods, especially high-fiber foods. No salt, no caffeine, no animal protein, no fried foods, no sugar, no white flour, no chocolate, no alcohol. Herbal remedies: kelp, garlic, dandelion root, alfalfa, horsetail, juniper berries, parsley.

EMPHYSEMA

Allopathic control: Oxygen, quit smoking.

Natural control: Stop smoking and take vitamins A, E, and C. Eat garlic and raw foods; but no meat, no eggs, no dairy, and no junk foods. Herbs: fenugreek, thyme, rosemary, mullein tea, aspidosperma.

GALLBLADDER DISEASE

Allopathic control: Low fat diet, surgery.

Natural control: Lemon juice and olive oil therapy. Increase fiber, avoid sugar, keep to a vegetarian diet, and lose weight. Cut out fat in diet; add vitamins C, E, essential fatty acids, and lecithin; check for food sensitivities; and check for low stomach acid.

GLAUCOMA

Allopathic control: Eye drops; surgery may help.

Natural control: Take vitamins A, thiamine, C, and bioflavonoids. Check for food sensitivities. Herbal remedies: Eyebright, golden seal, bayberry bark.

GOUT

Allopathic control: Avoid liver, take Allopurinal for control of uric acid.

Natural control: Take vitamins A, B-complex, folic acid, pantothenic acid, C and E; and calcium, magnesium, kelp, zinc. Try a strict diet of raw fruit and vegetable juices for two weeks, with no sugar, no white flour, and no animal protein. Herbal remedies: Cherry juice, celery juice, burdock, hyssop, juniper, birch.

HEART ATTACK (Coronary Artery Disease)

Allopathic control: Bed rest, streptokinase IV, oxygen, bypass surgery.

Natural control: Diet change: no fat, no sugar, no red meat, no caffeine, no alcohol, no tobacco, and no spicy foods. Homeopathy, vitamins A, B-complex, and C; minerals calcium, magnesium, and zinc; lecithin, garlic, selenium, methionine, cysteine. Herbs: Hawthorne berries, chickweed, cayenne, *Crataegus oxyacantha*, cactus grande, *Digitalis purpurea*, *Scilla maritima*, linden flower, *Ginkgo*.

HEARTBURN

Allopathic control: Antacids, rule out ulcer, hiatal hernia.

Natural control: No fried foods, fats, sugar, processed spicy food. Food sensitivity is a common cause. Herbal cures: Licorice root, slippery elm.

HEAVY METAL POISONING

Allopathic control: Chelation, avoidance.

Natural control: Diet change, increasing vitamins A, C, and B-complex; minerals zinc, calcium, magnesium, selenium, and manganese; and garlic, fiber, methionine, cysteine, glutathione, algin from sea plants like kelp; chelation.

HYPOCHONDRIASIS

Allopathic control: Reassurance, tonics.

Natural control: Homeopathy, bach flowers, counseling.

HYPOGLYCEMIA

Allopathic control: Deny there is such a condition.

Natural control: Five small meals a day, little sugar, no coffee, homeopathy. Take B-complex, pantothenic acid, C, raw adrenal, chromium, proteolytic enzymes, protein powder, calcium, royal jelly, carnitine, cysteine, and glutamine. No sugar, no junk food. Food allergies can cause low blood sugar.

IMPOTENCE

Allopathic control: Reassurance, psychiatry, control diabetes.

Natural control: Take vitamins B-complex and E, plus tyrosine, zinc, raw glandular complex, and GH_3. Diet: high protein, low fat, whole grains; and no junk food. Herbal remedies: Pumpkin seeds, bee pollen, ginseng, gotu kola, saw palmetto berries, damiana.

INFERTILITY

Allopathic control: Hormones, artificial insemination, surgery.

Natural control: No sugar; add zinc, B_6, C, and L-arginine.

INSOMNIA

Allopathic control: Sleeping pills, sleep clinic, psychiatry.

Natural control: Control stress. Change diet. Take calcium, tryptophan, B-complex, and C. No caffeine, alcohol, tobacco, or sugar. Homeopathy. Herbal remedies: Valerian root, hops, passion flower, skullcap, catnip, chamomille, valerian, *Avena sativa*.

IRRITABLE BOWEL SYNDROME

Allopathic control: Change diet, tranquilizers.

Natural control: Rule out food sensitivities and low stomach acid. Add dietary fiber, folic acid, lactobacillus, peppermint oil; no sugar.

KIDNEY STONES

Allopathic control: Surgery.

Natural control: No sugar, increase fiber, add magnesium, and stick to a vegetarian diet. Change minerals and supplements depending on type of stone.

MEMORY LOSS

Allopathic control: "Write things down."

Natural control: Take B_6, lecithin, pantothenic acid, niacin, C, glutamine, phenylalanine, GH_3, and choline. Change diet: eat small amounts frequently, no sugar, no junk food. Herbs: Rosemary, *Euphrasia rostokoviana*, *Salvia officinalis*, *Ginkgo*.

MÉNIÈRE'S SYNDROME (Tinnitus)

Allopathic control: Tranquilizers.

Natural control: Rule out aluminum and lead poisoning; control hypoglycemia; reduce fats and cholesterol; no sugar; add vitamins A, D, calcium, magnesium, zinc, manganese, bioflavonoids, niacin, B-complex, essential fatty acids.

MENOPAUSE

Allopathic control: Synthetic estrogen, tranquilizers.

Natural control: Check for low thyroid. Control hypoglycemia; rub natural progesterone cream on the skin. No stimulants, add vitamin E, lecithin, tryptophan, bioflavonoids, B_6, pantothenic acid, potassium, essential fatty acids, betaine HCl. Herbal remedies: Sage, ginseng, squaw vine, black cohosh, red raspberry, licorice, gotu kola, ginseng, kelp, *Vitex*, burdock, chamomilla, *Cimicifuga racemosa*.

MIGRAINE

Allopathic control: Cafergot, other pain medicines.

Natural control: Check for food sensitivities. No caffeine; add choline, essential fatty acids, niacinamide, rutin, pangamic acid, calcium, B-complex, C, pantothenic acid. Herbs: Feverfew, *Vinca major*.

MULTIPLE SCLEROSIS

Allopathic control: Low fat diet, wheelchair.

Natural control: Change to low-fat diet, no sugar, caffeine, to-bacco, or alcohol. Add essential fatty acids (linoleic acid was found to be low in the blood of MS patients), vitamins A, C, E, B-complex, inositol, choline, calcium, magnesium, potassium, manganese, phosphorus, sulfur, kelp, selenium, lecithin, digestive enzymes, and amino acids to improve the immune system. Rule out mercury poisoning. (Death rates from MS related to the numbers of decayed, missing, and filled teeth.)

MUSCLE ACHES

Allopathic control: Aspirin, acetaminophen, antispasmodics.

Natural control: Chiropractic care; add calcium, magnesium, vitamin E, and potassium. Useful herbs: *Arnica, Ruta, Hypericum, Cimicifuga*.

OBESITY

Allopathic control: Eat less. Cut out fat and cholesterol, exercise.

Natural control: Check for low thyroid and food sensitivities. Cut out fats and sugar; try a vegetarian diet, high in fiber, kelp, C, B_6, E, essential fatty acids, brewer's yeast, lecithin, amino acids, carnitine, phenylalanine. Try a three-day juice fast once a month. Exercise. Herbs: *Ficus*, yohimbe.

ODORS (Body)

Allopathic control: "Bathe more, use deodorants."

Natural control: Add magnesium; zinc may help. Cut out spicy foods. Control constipation; stop eating animal protein.

OSTEOPOROSIS

Allopathic control: Calcium, fluoride, estrogen, exercise.

Natural control: Use natural progesterone, calcium, magnesium, A, D (cod liver oil), C, boron, sulfur, silicon, and kelp. Exercise. Reduce animal protein. Herbs: Horsetail, shavegrass, oatstraw, nettles.

PARASITES

Allopathic control: Drugs for the specific parasite.

Natural control: Add herbs, garlic, onions, walnut shells, *Lactobacillus acidophilus*, *Spigelia*, and aspidium.

PREGNANCY

Allopathic control: Considered an abnormality. Gain only twenty to twenty-five pounds during the whole nine months, take a multiple vitamin, may need a Caesarian section.

Natural control: Gain twenty-five to thirty plus pounds. Take 2 to 5 grams of vitamin C a day, and extra vitamin B, calcium, and magnesium. Herbs: Raspberry leaves, nettles, alfalfa.

PREMENSTRUAL SYNDROME (PMS)

Allopathic control: Hormones, aspirin, exercise.

Natural control: Use B_6, magnesium, essential fatty acids, natural progesterone cream, vitamins A and E, kelp, calcium, and zinc. Exercise. No salt, caffeine, alcohol, smoking, red meats, dairy, sugar, or junk food. Herbs: *Rubus idaeus*, black cohosh root, licorice root, raspberry leaf, squaw vine, parsley.

PROSTATE HYPERTROPHY

Allopathic control: Surgery, rule out cancer.

Natural control: Rule out cancer. Use: Bee pollen; essential fatty acids; vitamins A, E, C, and B_6; zinc; magnesium; kelp; raw glandular prostate; and garlic. Avoid alcohol, sugar, coffee, and salt. Herbs: Pumpkin seeds, saw palmetto.

PSORIASIS

Allopathic control: Drugs.

Natural control: Use vitamins A, E, and C; magnesium; lecithin; B-complex; folic acid; B$_{12}$; zinc; essential fatty acids; and proteolytic enzymes. Stop meat, dairy, sugar, junk food. Eat 50 percent raw diet. Herbs: Dandelion, goldenseal, yellow dock, sarsaparilla, burdock.

SLIPPED DISC

Allopathic control: Surgery.

Natural control: Braces, chiropractic manipulation.

STOMACHACHES

Allopathic control: Rule out appendicitis and ulcer. Antispasmodics, antacids.

Natural control: Rule out need for surgery. Change diet, no milk, wheat, eggs, or nuts. (See Dyspepsia.) Herbs: *Mentha*, *Ulmus*, *Althea*, licorice root.

STROKE (see also Hypertension)

Allopathic control: Rest and rehabilitation: learn to use walker; control blood pressure.

Natural control: Change diet, more potassium (vegetables).

ULCERS

Allopathic control: Antacids, stop smoking, drugs.

Natural control: Add vitamins A, E, and B-complex; zinc; aloe vera; fiber; plus drink carrot and cabbage juice daily. No tobacco, caffeine, alcohol, fried foods, spices. Herbal remedies: *Orzya sativa*, *Panicum miliaceum*, *Triticum vulgare*, licorice root, slippery elm.

VISION PROBLEMS

Allopathic control: Drops for glaucoma, surgery for crossed eyes and cataracts.

Natural control: Developmental optometrists, training. Herb: Blueberry.

WARTS

Allopathic control: Liquid nitrogen, surgery.

Natural control: Vitamin A: 100,000 units daily for seven to ten days.

These various therapies are compatible with the Life Balances program. They can be used simultaneously. It is expected that the L.B. program will allow clients to reduce the reliance on other therapies. People who have consistently stuck with the program will notice improvement in weeks; sometimes in months. Most will then relax a little. They will go through the smelling kit only two or three times a week and take their blood pressure but twice a week. They might get their blood analyzed only once or twice a year. A new symptom or a flu bug striking means a "shingle has blown off the roof," and a little repair work is necessary. The electrolyte solution that has been formulated by Mr. Kitkoski is worth using daily and especially in hot weather and if stressed more than that. I ran out of mine last week, had some ice cream the other night, and awakened with a killer calf-cramp.

13

Electrolytes: Another Sine Qua Non of Life

If I asked you what you considered the most important organ in your body, you might simply say, "My heart." An intellectual type might want the brain to have that honor. A macho Rambo-type might feel if his you-know-what were to disappear, he'd die. Someone observing the seeming endless guillotining during the French Revolution remarked, "The head and the body must be interdependent, as they both die when separated." (The start of psychosomatic medicine?)

Everything in the body is connected in some way or another with every other part. Your brain tells your little toe to move. Cheese in your stomach now will give your bones some calcium in a few hours. Blood is more than just water carrying red cells and oxygen to all the cells of the body. (About 65 to 70 percent of the body's weight is H_2O.) In order for us to live and function that blood must carry dissolved minerals. These are called electrolytes: compounds that, when dissolved, dissociate into charged particles, called ions. These create an electrical charge, like a battery. So the most important factor that keeps us alive is electricity. The human body is like a machine and runs on these positive and negative ions. Without electrolytes and the electricity they produce, life is impossible.

Some ions, called cations, are positively charged: sodium $(Na+)$, potassium $(K+)$, calcium $(Ca++)$, and magnesium $(Mg++)$. The negatively charged ions are anions: chloride $(Cl-)$, bicarbonate (HCO_3-), and phosphate $(HPO_4=)$. Plain water does not conduct an electric current, but when these compounds are dissolved in water, as in our blood, the fluid can then conduct a current. Apparently living things need this current; it may, in fact, be our soul.

Buffering Capacity

Electrolytes in the blood serve to maintain the acid/base balance by buffering the acidic and alkaline elements. They help to maintain the proper volume of blood so the blood pressure is adequate to circulate the blood to all parts. This electrolyte solution acts as a carrying agent for some amino acids and minerals. The fluid is as important as the dissolved salts *in* the blood. These elements in the body need to be in balance for the systems to function at full capacity. If the amounts of these specific ions are not in the proper ratios, it will affect general health and blood pressure. Any electrolytic solution of any concentration contains the same number of mEqs of anions as cations. It's the law. We are constantly losing these electrolytes from the body and if they are not replaced in the proper amounts and ratios, some symptom or disease appears to remind us. You must keep the little batteries charged. Not too little and not too much.

Many athletes feel that consuming sports drinks, like Gatorade, improves their performance. But research going back to 1969 indicates that moderate electrolyte loss from moderate exercise can be compensated for by ordinary food. Excessive salt loss from heavy exercise can be balanced with ordinary salt tablets and plenty of water. The body conserves sodium energetically with an efficient homeostatic mechanism; our ancestors evolved on a diet low in sodium and high in potassium. Nowadays, we need less sodium than potassium.

Intracellular and Extracellular

The cellular membrane separates the intracellular and extracellular compartments and has many functions, one of which is to permit the free movement of water molecules. The difference in the solute concentrations is explained by a pump (sodium pump), in constant operation in the cell wall to push the sodium out of the cell and keep the potassium in. If it were not for this pump, the concentration of the particles would be the same in and out of the cells. The body's cells apparently need more potassium than sodium. But many people ingest more sodium than potassium; it can explain, in part, why they are fatigued and have high blood pressure. If more sodium than potassium is ingested, the sodium pump slows. A calcium pump is also slowed. Calcium then enters the cells and the increased muscle tension of the blood vessel walls increases the blood pressure.

If we eat properly with plenty of fruits and vegetables, shouldn't we get enough of these electrolytes? How are we losing them? The body has some of these electrolytes stored, but they are not just hanging around like our fat storage depots. We can lose them rapidly if we exercise in hot weather, if we get a high fever, or especially if we develop vomiting and diarrhea. All doctors have had patients who were recovering from a sickness and then suddenly, and inexplicably, die. If some alert intern happened to see the "lytes" blood panel, the results might have shown a distorted balance or skewed ratios of the electrolytes, especially the sodium and the potassium.

Dehydration/Overhydration

I recall a child who was dehydrated with elevated concentrations of all the electrolytes. I gave him a rapid intravenous drip of a diluted salt solution because his sodium was very high (150 mEq/L). He needed water. When about 100 cc had run in, he had a seizure and became limp and stuporous. His sodium level at that time was about 140, but the fluid had run in too fast. The electrolyte gradient from the intracellular nerve cell concentration was too much for the extracellular concentration and an electrical imbalance triggered the seizure. The appropriate intravenous solution brought him around.

One can see how interdependent the functions of the body are upon the relative concentrations of the different constituents of the blood and the extra- and intra-cellular compartments.

If a person drinks more plain water than his body needs, he may experience water intoxication. The water is absorbed into the plasma of the blood, increasing the blood volume and the blood pressure. This forces water into the extra- or inter-cellular compartment. The concentration of the sodium chloride in the extracellular space will drop and abnormal amounts of water will flow into the cells by simple diffusion. It is called excessive cellular hydration.

The maintenance and balance of the water content of the plasma depends upon the blood pressure and the plasma protein concentration, as in the following examples of osmotic pressure:

If a person continues on a low-protein or starvation diet, the plasma protein level will drop. Water moves from the plasma to the extracellular compartment, leading to edema and a swollen belly.

If a person is dehydrated, the loss of water from the plasma will create a relative increase in protein concentration, and water is taken from the extracellular department.

We have all heard of desperate people who, trying to lose weight, went on a high protein, low fruit, low vegetable, and low grain diet. Unable to conserve potassium over the period of this dietary restriction, they died because of a heart arrhythmia, a fairly common condition if the serum potassium reaches a low level.

Crazy, unbalanced diets with either too much water or not enough of the essential salts that make these electrolytes lead inevitably to sickness, and, as we can see, even death.

Fluid Intake

Water intake is critical. The amount of water taken in during an average day should be about two to three liters. Imbibed water amounts to about one to 1½ liters, and the rest comes from the water contained in foods. (Vegetables are about 90 percent water.) Good health can be achieved only when the balance of water and electrolytes is optimal. The body tries to correct imbalances but can only do so if adequate amounts of water, protein, and the salts are ingested. If one has low blood pressure, sodium will be absorbed at a faster rate than the potassium. Potassium is absorbed more readily than sodium in those with high blood pressure. Drinking a fluid with all the necessary electrolytes is the best way to maintain the fluid and electrolyte balance. Electrolytes and water are lost constantly via the kidneys, sweat glands, and the intestines. Drinking water is a good idea, but fluids with electrolytes would be a better replacement plan, especially during heavy exercise and hot weather.

If electrolytes are not supplied in adequate amounts, the kidneys try to compensate. The total sodium excreted in the urine for each twenty-four hour period is about the same as the sodium intake, which obviously varies with the diet. The range for sodium excretion is about three to eight grams a day, and varies inversely with the potassium output. Aldosterone, an adrenal cortical hormone, stimulates the kidneys to reabsorb sodium and reject the potassium. (This hormone is produced when there is stress, dehydration, or hemorrhage, so that the sodium and increased fluid that accompanies it will help increase the blood pressure.)

Without water, there can be no life. Blood, lymph, digestive juices, urine, sweat, and tears use water as a solvent to transport nutrients. Water is needed to carry wastes out of the body. Embryos and the brain are cushioned in a watery environment. Sound and light waves are transmitted to eyes and ears via watery media.

Many people fail to respond to the sensation of thirst: the dry mouth. If the total fluid in the body, blood, and extracellular compartments is not sufficient to carry the nutrients to all the cells and return with the waste products, the vascular system will respond with a generalized constriction of the arterioles, venules, and capillaries. The body is smart enough to maintain the blood supply to the lungs, the heart, the liver, and the kidneys to maintain life. Then one notices cold hands and feet. When the fluid level is down as indicated by the constricted veins in the arms, legs, and head, the victim tires easily due to lack of oxygen in the system. He is more likely to have headaches. It is the beginning of other diseases, the result of poor circulation. Tension in the shoulders and neck is a good example of this. Picture a plastic jug, partially filled with water. If you squeeze the sides of the jug, the water level rises. This is what happens in your body when veins constrict to compensate for lack of fluid. This also explains why you might feel dizzy when you arise too rapidly: There is not enough blood circulating to your head and your sense of balance is off.

Fluid Level

Do this little test right now: While seated, place your hand, palm down, on your thigh. The veins on the back of your hand should stand up above the surface and feel moderately firm and puffy. If your veins are full, slowly raise your hand and watch when the veins collapse. They should be able to carry some blood in them until they reach your eye level. If they become flat at your nipple level, you are really low in fluid, maybe a quart down. If the veins collapse at your chin level you are a pint low. At those levels you should be able to say, "Yes, I am thirsty." You would also notice that your hands and feet are cold. (If the veins stay full when your hand is above your head, you may be in heart failure. See your doctor. If your veins are not up when your hand is on your leg, your fluid level is very low and your electrolytes are out of balance.)

The fluid level must be higher than the level of your heart in order to provide proper circulation to all parts of your body. The fluid level must be great enough to transport toxins from your system. Normal wear and tear, but especially injuries and exercise, will deposit garbage about the body. If this material stays in the tissues, healing cannot begin. If you damage cells and the proper materials are not available for repair, that cell or group of cells will die. Proper circulation plus a balanced chemistry will deliver the necessary new material and replace the damaged cells, and remove the unhealthy, waste materials. The electrolytes help to flush out the waste materials.

When this unhealthy material is picked up by the circulation, it travels around the body and when it flows through the brain, it may make a person feel bad, so some people shun water. But there is no other way to get rid of wastes.

When your fluid level is up, your skin will feel warm and moist to the touch and will have elasticity and turgor. If the sodium level is high, the veins are usually up. (See Rambo in the movies: huge muscles with the veins in his arms standing out about ready to pop. He may have a stroke any day.)

We need water, but not too much or we wash out the good things along with the garbage.

The work of Dr. Sidney Ringer showed that the best replacement fluid is that which most closely imitates the electrolyte concentration of the serum. The ratios of the calcium, sodium, and potassium in Ringer's solution are at the proper physiological concentration so that when this solution is orally consumed or provided intravenously, the blood pressure will be neither raised nor lowered.

Some people crave certain soft drinks. They are fluid, so they can be helpful, but the artificial sugars, the phosphates, and the caffeine in so many of them make them worthless. Although coffee and tea are fluids, the caffeine in them tends to act as a diuretic, and the imbiber may lose more fluid than gained. Alcohol has a similar stimulating effect on the kidneys; the net effect is a loss of fluid from the body. Diet 7UP may be all right for some people who know that they are alkaline and need the carbonate, but a carbonated seltzer water is better. When you drink just water, you constantly dilute the amount of nutrients in your body; water acts as a diuretic.

I remember a sixty-year-old woman who had X-radiation to her mouth and salivary glands for cancer therapy. She produced no saliva, so to alleviate her dry mouth she sipped on water all day (about three quarts a day). She was weak, tired, and forgetful. Her blood test showed she was at the low end of the normal range for sodium and chloride. A solution like Ringer's to sip on brought her health almost to normal.

The best thing to do is to get your blood tested, at least the electrolyte panel: the sodium, potassium, the CO_2, and the chloride. If you are low in sodium (below 140 mEq/L) you are more likely to have low blood pressure, a low fluid level, and cold hands and feet. Many vegetarians are thus because the fruits and vegetables they eat metabolize into vinegar (acetic acid) in the body and this takes sodium out of the system via the kidneys and lowers the pressure.

If your sodium is above 142 mEq/L, you are more likely to have elevated blood pressure, enlarged veins on your arms and hands, and warm hands and feet. You probably like vinegar, and it is safe for you to drink it as long as it tastes good to you. If the results of the blood test show you have a high concentration of nutrients due to low fluid intake, you need to drink an electrolyte solution.

I met a lady who had cold hands and feet, frequent headaches, and a sallow complexion. She had to wear socks to bed, and sometimes gloves; her sex life was nil, and life was a drag.

"Stress," she was told by her doctor. Her blood test revealed nutrient deficiencies, and low amounts of electrolyte, especially the sodium (down to 137 mEq/L). We had her drink three glasses of electrolyte mixed half and half with milk daily. In ten days, her headaches were gone, her hands warmed up, and her low blood pressure moved up to a normal 120 over 70. She felt great and even had a date for the next weekend.

It is important to find out if calcium is in the ionized or nonionized state. Electrolyte trouble arises when the ionized form is converted to the nonionized form due to a state of alkalosis. (The ionized form of calcium should always be higher than the calcium.) Alkalosis can be determined by subtracting the acidic elements (CO_2 + chloride) from the alkaline elements (sodium + potassium). The answer should be between 6 and 12. If it is higher, and 80 percent of the population in North America show those higher figures, then the calcium may not be in the ionized form and muscle cramps and paresthesias may result. If the calcium is on the low side, the electrolytes are usually consumed mixed half and half with 2 percent milk, two to three times a day. This will balance the electrolytes, increase the fluid level by increasing the circulation, and will flush out the waste materials from the body. Good health is the result of a balance of water and electrolytes. A scientifically formulated electrolyte replacement drink is your best method of maintaining a healthy internal environment.

Don't be rude to your body; it's the only one you get.

Skip This if Chemistry is Unfriendly to You

Experience has proven that the best way to express the concentration of these electrolytes is in terms of milliequivalents per liter (mEq/L). A milliequivalent is the amount of one ion that will exactly react with or replace a mEq of another ion. E.g., 1 mEq of Na + will exactly react with one mEq of Cl − ; 2 mEq of K + will exactly react with 2 mEq of HCO_3 − .

If one adds a pinch of salt, a bit of $NaHCO_3$, a few granules of K_2SO_4, and a little $CaCl_2$ to a glass of water, the total mEq of the cations (Na + ,K + ,Ca + +) would equal the total mEq of the anions (HCO_3 − ,SO_4 = ,and Cl −).

The 24 chemical screen blood-test measures the serum electrolytes in the three types of body fluids: the *extracellular fluid*, which consists of both *plasma* (blood) and the *intercellular fluid* (fluid between cells), and the *intracellular fluid* (the fluid inside cells). The intercellular fluid is similar in its ionic pattern to the blood, but the protein concentrations are very different: 16 mEq/L in the plasma and but 1 mEq/L in the intercellular fluid. (Proteins are considered anions.) The sodium (Na) is 142, the potassium (K) and calcium (Ca) are 5 mEq/L each, and the magnesium (Mg) is 2 mEq/L. Anions: chloride (Cl) is usually 103, bicarbonate (HCO_3) is 27, phosphate (HPO_4) is 2 mEq/L, and other organic acids are about 6. The total concentrations of anions and cations in the serum approximates 154 to 155 mEq/L.

The concentration of the electrolytes inside the cells (intracellular) varies considerably from their concentration on the outside (extracellular). The concentration of the potassium inside the cell is up to 160 mEq/L, while it is but 5 on the outside. The sodium inside is only 10 (outside = 142), and the chloride is but 3 (outside it is 103).

There are three Life Balances electrolyte formulae. They all have the dissolved nutrients to supply the proper balance, but one has more sodium in it for those with low blood pressure and a low sodium level. Another has less sodium for those with elevated blood pressure and who carry a high amount of sodium in their blood. The third has a normal amount of sodium for those who need the electrolytes, but have a normal blood pressure and a reasonably normal level of sodium in their blood.

14

Hypertension: The Silent Killer

I would hope in some small way to get the message out to the public that there are better ways to control blood pressure, either high or low, than just using drugs. It would be nice if the medical profession took a closer look at this chapter and try to implement some of the universal laws of chemistry so drug use would be knocked down to the bottom of the choice list. The cooperation of the patient is absolutely necessary. But the patient *and* the doctor should work together—the doctor monitoring the blood pressure—the patient eating properly and taking the necessary supplements. There is no doubt that most all blood pressure abnormalities can be controlled with diet and supplements. However, we want to confront the causes and not just the symptoms. If one has a stone in his shoe, he should remove the stone and not just take more aspirin for the pain.

Medical Therapy

Medical therapy, encouraged by the pharmaceutical industry, has taken the responsibility of disease control *away* from the patient. Total health care moved to the doctor's hands, and, consequently, a whole generation has grown up dependent upon the allopathic physician. Recently patients have begun to ask why they get sick. They no longer like the idea of just taking drugs to mask symptoms and signs. They want to discover the cause of the infirmity and eliminate it.

I have learned in the last few years that the body can be relied upon to seek its own adjustment to homeostasis and normality. Sickness, I now understand, means that there is a tilt in the body's chemistry. Climate, stressors, poor diet, injuries can all trigger a change in the delicate balance of the fluids and minerals, and, consequently, a disease appears. Because everyone is different in genetic and chemical makeup, not everyone will get the same sickness. If one makes some basic and safe adjustment in nutrient intake, one can return to normal functioning, usually without medication, no matter what the name of the disease.

So it is with blood pressure control.

We need blood to live, and we need enough pressure to push the blood through the vessels—not too much and not too little. Humans were not meant to have such low pressure that they feel cold and tired, nor have high blood pressure and die of a stroke. There are a variety of feedback mechanisms—mainly chemical ratios—in the body to bring the pressure up when it is too low and to lower it when it is too high. But if the proper amounts of vitamins and minerals and fluid are not available to the body, these buffering functions of the physiology are not adequate to keep the body from sickness.

Causes of Hypertension

For decades scientists have been searching for the causes of high blood pressure, which the American Heart Association estimates afflicts more than 60 million Americans. More than 500,000 Americans will have a stroke this year, and of that group, 150,000 will die. Fifty percent of the population over age 50 years probably has high blood pressure. In time even those people with mildly elevated blood pressure will develop a thickening of the walls of the small arteries and arterioles in their kidneys. The cause is unknown in 90 percent of the cases, hence the name: "essential hypertension." We now know that these "unknown" causes of hypertension are really imbalances in the ratios of the electrolytes and minerals in the bloodstream.

These are the factors known to affect the pressure:
1) Age: Older people are more likely to have elevated pressure;
2) Race: African–Americans are more susceptible to hypertension;
3) Sex: Males are more likely to have elevated blood pressure.
Other causes include obesity, sodium sensitivity, alcohol ingestion (which may raise the blood pressure in some), oral contraceptives (they have been known to affect some women), and lack of exercise.

The cutoff point for systolic pressure has been set at 140 mm of mercury; above this value doctors advise patients to "watch it." If the pressure climbs to 150 and especially 160 mm, the doctor usually prescribes some drug that will reduce the systolic (upper reading) pressure, but may not affect the diastolic (lower reading).

The diastolic pressure is the amount of consistent pressure expressed in mm of mercury that continues to push the blood through the vessels in between the beats of the heart. It is supposed to be around 80. Seventy-five to 85 is about right. If that diastolic pressure is sustained above 90, doctors get nervous and want to prescribe something, usually a diuretic that removes sodium from the body. It does work, but it also takes potassium from the system and potassium is the very element that the body needs to keep the lower, diastolic pressure at that safe level of around 80.

Dr. Sidney Ringer

Dr. Sidney Ringer, whom we mentioned in previous chapters, checked the response of the heart and vascular system to various chemicals in the blood. He found that in the frog, if a saline (salt or sodium chloride) solution was dripped onto the open heart of the frog, the heart stopped in a tetanic contraction, like a chronic systole. He rightly assumed that elevated blood pressure was a function of too much sodium in the blood. This was a partial answer. He also found that if the exposed heart of the frog was perfused with a potassium solution, the heart would stop in a relaxed or diastolic position. Therefore, he concluded, extra sodium raises the systolic pressure, and extra potassium lowers the diastolic pressure.

Other researchers have found that calcium, magnesium, water, hormones, alcohol, and other elements in the blood affect pressure. Blood pressure control is the response of the heart and the blood vessels to a variety of elements in the blood and to the physiology of the body.

Blood pressure is a function of the total systemic blood flow pushing against the resistance offered by the blood vessels, mainly the arterioles. The kidneys participate as *they* affect peripheral resistance and blood volume. Through rather complicated feedback mechanisms the kidney produces vasopressor and vaso-depressor agents; these mainly work by conserving or releasing water and reabsorbing or excreting sodium.

Hypotension

If there is a drop in the circulating arterial volume, such as after a heavy hemorrhage, receptor cells in the kidneys produce an enzyme, called renin, which acts upon angiotensinogen, synthesized by the liver and angiotensin I is formed. As this latter peptide passes through the lungs, angiotensin II is formed. This one stimulates the adrenal glands to produce aldosterone, which promotes sodium reabsorption that will prevent the reduction of the circulating arterial volume. Blood pressure is maintained at the optimal level. Newly discovered renal prostaglandins affect the blood pressure. It is to be remembered that the total body sodium is the main determinant of extracellular fluid volume, and the kidneys are the principal organs responsible for sodium homeostasis. But salt restriction alone is an ineffective means of controlling blood pressure. As is the case with most things in the body, a ratio is involved. So with blood pressure, the ratio of the sodium to the potassium is the determining factor: *The proportion of each element balances the blood pressure.* One can have high blood pressure with normal sodium and low potassium.

Like most everything involving humans, essential high blood pressure is a combination of genetic and environmental factors. It has been *proven* so in comparative studies with twins, siblings, families, African–Americans, much of the populations of the U.S., Europe, and Japan. When the salt intake rises to 10 grams a day (two teaspoonfuls) as in the U.S., there is an incidence of hypertension approaching 25 percent or so, regardless of genetic factors. The more salt, the greater the percent of the population is affected. In some parts of Japan where the salt intake reaches 35 grams, it is amazing that not all the adults have hypertension. A 20 percent minority may have a genetic resistance.

Thus high blood pressure does run in families, but it is difficult to separate shared genetic factors from shared lifestyles, as families continue to eat the same diet through the generations. Families repeat the same meals every ten days or so and recipes are passed on from one generation to another. It's true that what we eat is what we are.

The susceptibility of individuals to hypertension depends more on the amount of acetic acid (vinegar) available to the kidneys. This acid removes sodium from the body. Excess alkalinity is more of a threat to the individual than the sodium as it relates to causing high blood pressure.

Those who eat fish, meat, and salads with vinegar dressings (acidic foods), have a low systolic pressure. A runner's blood pressure is usually around $110/60$, because exercise causes a loss of sodium via the sweat and the urine. The sodium is lost, but the potassium is conserved by the kidneys. The sodium/potassium ratio is lowered. These runners *must* run to provide their bodies with circulation to feel good. At rest with that low level of pressure, their hearts cannot pump enough blood to circulate an adequate volume. As long as the person continues to have a low sodium intake and continues to exercise, the blood pressure will continue to drop or at least to stay too low for health.

We have all met the thin, neurasthenia, washed-out person who continues to have the "vapors"—weak and always fatigued. He is not anemic, but his blood pressure is low (110 over 60), hands and feet are cold (he may have to wear socks to bed), his bowels are sluggish (constipation), and everything points to a low thyroid condition. His veins are small and it is difficult to extract blood for testing.

These people thus afflicted have low sodium levels, and they are more likely to get every infection that comes along. They may have a high cholesterol level (above 275 mg per dl), which tends to make the low thyroid theory a valid one. But the high cholesterol is more likely due to the low pulse pressure that is unable to push the blood through the vessels with sufficient force to clean out the cholesterol.

Vegan–Vegetarians with Low Blood Pressure

Many of these people are vegan–vegetarians (no dairy and no animal protein). They tend to have low blood pressure because the diet is high in the foods that turn to acetic acid, and as we have seen, acetic acid pulls sodium out of the tissues and when the sodium falls, so does the blood pressure. Along with the low blood pressure, fatigue, cold hands and feet, these people are susceptible to infections. It is common for them to be nutrient-deficient: low in calcium, magnesium, iron, and other essential elements. If there is a genetic tendency to elevated high blood pressure, it is more likely to be associated with the big muscular types (Rambo). As might be expected, their favorite foods are the salty, fatty ones. If these people have high-sodium and low-vinegar diets, they will have an elevated systolic pressure, but if they eat a well-rounded diet, including fruits and vegetables, and put vinegar on their daily salads, they will be able to reduce their sodium and keep the blood pressure under some control, even getting it down to a normal level.

Some researchers feel it is an immunity problem. Certain chemicals irritate the muscles in the arterioles and constrict them more than necessary to maintain an adequate pressure. People who tend to have more alkaline fluids than acidic ones are more likely to have elevated blood pressure. Women who take extra calcium to avoid the ravages of osteoporosis, are setting themselves up for elevated blood pressure and a stroke rather than a fall and a broken hip.

Accumulation of data reveals a number of things. There is a direct relationship of C and calcium, which regulates the viscosity of the blood. Near the equator where the year-round warm temperature provides sunshine and lots of vegetation, the plants have a high concentration of vitamin C and vinegar. These acids, ascorbic and acetic, make the minerals, calcium, magnesium, zinc, phosphorus soluble and usable. The blood, therefore, becomes more acidic and thicker. The blood pressure tends to be lower. In the northern climes, with less sunshine and less vegetation, the C and the acetic acid are less abundant, and the calcium increases. The blood tends to become more alkaline and thinner. The BP becomes higher.

In the last fifty years the increased intake of sodium has caused an increase in height and an increase in blood pressure in many members of the population. We also are seeing many people with very low blood pressure because of the higher consumption of vegetables. The final product of vegetable metabolism in the body is vinegar. This removes sodium from their bodies. They tend to have lower blood pressure and smaller bones. Not everyone, therefore, should follow the recommendation of the American Heart Association and reduce their intake of salt. Everyone needs to have some salt in their diet, especially those with low blood pressure. When salt is restricted or eliminated from the diet, people tend to have more infections and bone disorders.

When milk is eliminated from the diet the result is an abnormal imbalance of calcium, phosphorus, and magnesium, which affects the circulation. Long-term calcium restriction is shown by no visible veins and poor circulation. Long-term and heavy use of milk is shown by protruding veins and hypertension.

Therefore, moderate ingestion of salt and milk with adequate vitamin C and vinegar results in general good health and circulation. It is almost impossible to eat enough of the right things to keep a proper chemical balance in the system—unless you know what you need. Proper eating of all types of food does more to correct the problems than therapy with medication.

Standard medicine has learned a few things about the treatment of elevated blood pressure: lose weight, cut down on the sodium, exercise, and increase the potassium-bearing foods. A chemical law might operate here: "The greater the concentration, the greater the rate of the reaction." If you have restricted your daily salt intake to no more than ⅔ of a teaspoon all your life, you will not have hypertension. If you have had hypertension for years, it may take a severe restriction down to just two pinches a day to lower your blood pressure. But if you restrict your sodium unduly, without a blood test to measure where your level is, you may do yourself some harm.

Drug Therapy

If the above diet and lifestyle changes are ineffective, doctors reach for the prescription pad. Diuretics are their first choice as these drugs increase the elimination of salt (potassium and sodium) and water, causing mild dehydration and reducing the blood volume. They may cause an increase in cholesterol and the blood sugar, however.

If that is not effective, beta-blockers are added. These drugs dampen the heart's pumping action. They may cause fatigue and impotence.

Then it is to the ACE inhibitors. They block the angiotensin converting enzyme so blood pressure is lowered. Expensive.

Calcium channel blockers relax the arterial wall muscles. Expensive.

The side effects from these drugs could be avoided if the rules of chemistry are followed. Each person must learn to make proper choices, not just cover up the problem with medication. An individual regulating his own blood pressure must make sure that the doctor is held accountable. You must not assume, for instance, that you have high sodium because you have high blood pressure. It may be alkalinity from calcium or other elements in the blood. A proper blood test, shared with the patient, can show the need for restricting salt or calcium, or show the doctor that the sodium and calcium are normal, so some other approach to the problem is needed.

Safe Experiments

HERE IS AN EXPERIMENT:

First, take your blood pressure and write down the numbers. Systolic (top)/diastolic (bottom) It should be about 120–135 (top or systolic)/75–85 (bottom or diastolic). Now, add a teaspoon of vinegar (white distilled is preferable) to an eight-ounce glass of water. Taste the vinegar water, and if you have a high systolic pressure (over 140) and the sodium in your blood test is elevated somewhat, the vinegar will taste mild. The higher the systolic pressure, the milder the vinegar flavor will be. It should taste like water if your systolic is 160 mm Hg or above.

But if you have a low systolic pressure (110 or lower), the vinegar will taste sour or even bitter. You are probably one who restricts salt in your diet or you eat a lot of vegetables and, as a consequence, you are making your own vinegar; this diet has removed sodium from your system already. You don't need to drink the vinegar water if it doesn't taste good. Your body is telling you that you do not need it; you have enough already. (It is even possible that your urine may test alkaline because the sodium coming out from the kidneys makes the urine alkaline. Vinegar, an acid, may make the body excrete an alkaline chemical.)

TRY THIS:

Add ⅛ teaspoon of sodium bicarbonate to an eight-ounce glass of distilled water. Sodium bicarbonate will always cause the systolic value to rise and will always make the space between the systolic and the diastolic wider.

HERE'S ONE:

Add ⅛ teaspoon of sodium chloride (table salt) to an eight-ounce glass of distilled water. Mix well and taste. NaCL will always cause the systolic to rise and will always make the space between the systolic and the diastolic wider apart. If it tastes thick, or okay, you need it; it tastes thin and very salty, you do not need it.

ANOTHER TEST:

Add ⅛ teaspoon of magnesium sulfate (Epsom salt) to an eight-ounce glass of distilled water. Mix well and taste. $MgSO_4$ will always cause your systolic and diastolic values to be closer together. If it tastes thick and sweet, you need it; if it tastes thin and sharp, or bitter, you do not need it.

TRY ONE MORE:

Add ⅛ teaspoon of potassium chloride to an eight-ounce glass of distilled water. Mix well and taste. Potassium chloride will always cause the diastolic value to lower, and the space between the systolic and the diastolic to be farther apart. If it tastes thick or good, you need it; if it tastes thin or bitter or salty, you do not need it.

The above examples indicate the methodology of how the chemistry of the body will indicate to the owner of the body how self-selection really works. It is based on the unignorable rules of chemistry. If an individual is taught to recognize his needs, and if his choices are proper, he can maintain a balanced chemistry.

Here are some seeming paradoxes. If an individual is high in sodium, he will crave salt. Someone who avoids salt creates a sodium/potassium imbalance, which makes the individual *dislike* salt. With a normal sodium/potassium ratio, which controls the nervous system, salt changes taste as an individual's need increases or decreases with intake.

Low sodium in a blood test shows a true level; there is no sodium stored in the body to be used by the system. It must be replaced, as it cannot be drawn from the kidneys if it is not there. Individuals with high sodium need to have their chemistry evaluated so they may understand their needs.

Physical and emotional illnesses develop when people have imbalances in their chemistry. Each individual is unique as the chemistry so clearly shows. Without the ability to measure and quantify chemical reactions and potentials, the field of medicine will remain an art, and never become a science. It is time for a specific accountable program that educates and makes each and every individual responsible.

We don't know everything, but we sure know how to look it up.

A Case Study
A Client with High Blood Pressure

INTERACTIONS WITH THE LIFE BALANCES HEALTH PROGRAM

Abstract A white female in her early fifties, diagnosed with both severe diastolic hypertension and isolated systolic hypertension (as defined by American Medical Association) was referred to Life Balances for evaluation. Her physicians were unable to control the blood pressure using medications or behavioral techniques (i.e., diet, reduction of salt intake, and/or relaxation techniques). Her initial blood pressure reading, for the first three days on the Life Balances Health Program was 161/107 (A.M.). After twelve months on the program her A.M. blood pressure was 139/90 and represents a decrease of 13 percent. Her initial P.M. blood pressure reading, for the first three days was 161/105 (P.M.). After twelve months on the program her P.M. blood pressure was 126/73. This represents a decrease of 26 percent. Given the lack of efficacy of any and all other treatments to reduce her blood pressure in the previous twenty-plus years, much of the change can be attributed

(continued on page 163)

(continued from page 162)

to the program. Further study of other clients reveals a similar success correlated to the proportion the individual used the program.

Report The client began the Life Balances Health Program on June 13, 1988. She had chronic high blood pressure, with diastolic readings over 100 mm/hg and systolic over 150 for the preceding years, anti-hypertensive medication had minimal effectiveness. The client was referred to Life Balances by a friend on the program. The woman contacted her physician and asked him to monitor her progress.

The average blood pressure for the client the first three days on the program was 161/107 (A.M.) (a mean of 134) and 161/105 (P.M.) (a mean of 133). She was given a standard regimen using the Life Balances Health Program that consisted of vitamins, minerals and electrolytes. Also, the client was educated to realize that a change in behavior patterns is important to improve her health. One of the program's goals is to educate the client to be a wise consumer and take more responsibility for personal health decisions. Six months after starting the Life Balances Health Program the client's average blood pressure for a two–week period was 139/95 (A.M.) (a mean of 117) and 131/84 (P.M.) (a mean of 108). This represents a decrease of 13 percent in the A.M. mean blood pressure and a 19 percent drop in the P.M. mean blood pressure. Three years later her A.M. blood pressure was 133/88 (a mean of 111) and the P.M. blood pressure was 119/80 (a mean of 108). This represents a total drop in blood pressure of 17 percent in A.M. readings and 25 percent in P.M. readings and shows the long-term effects of the program. Also the client was able to successfully discontinue taking the high blood pressure medications with their inherent side effects.

During the past year the client has spent an average of $56.76 per month (at Life Balances) to maintain her health. In addition to her improvement in blood pressure readings, she was able to report an improvement in her attitude as well as a greater ability to control her health problems. Her physician has acknowledged her improvement at each annual checkup.

The accompanying graphs show the definitive evidence of the clients gradual lowering of blood pressure (systolic and diastolic A.M. and P.M.). This was for the 12-month period after starting the program. In this instance, the client was able to supply us with a wealth of data, including blood pressure readings each A.M. and P.M. for over three years (still ongoing). This is indicative of almost all clients on the Life Balances Health Program.

(continued on page 164)

(continued from page 163)

Figure 1: Systolic Pressure (A.M.)

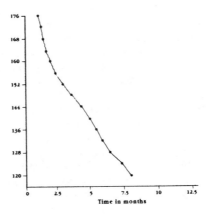

Each point represents an actual A.M. systolic blood pressure reading.

Figure 2: Diastolic Pressure (A.M.)

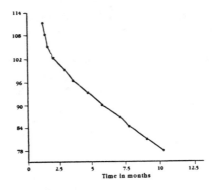

Each point represents an actual A.M. diastolic blood pressure reading.

(continued on page 165)

(continued from page 164)

Figure 3: Systolic Pressure (P.M.)

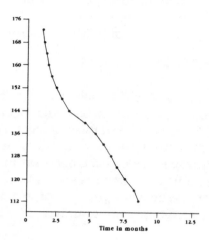

Each point represents an actual P.M. systolic blood pressure reading.

Figure 4: Diastolic Pressure (P.M.)

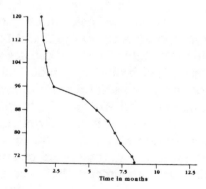

Each point represents an actual P.M. diastolic blood pressure reading.

Hypertension

Natural control of elevated blood pressure that naturopathic physicians might use includes a vegetarian diet, no salt, vitamin B-complex, choline, inositol, C, E, calcium, magnesium, lecithin, potassium, zinc, selenium, fiber, octacosanol, kelp, garlic, cratagus berry, linden flowers, mistletoe.

Here is the story of a woman with low blood pressure:

LOW BLOOD PRESSURE

C. J. is a forty-seven-year-old female investor/secretary, 5 feet 7 inches, 168 pounds. Her blood pressure has been hovering down at 96/72 to 95/56. Her chief complaints are chronic depression, loss of short-term memory, a short attention span, and exhaustion. She took Prozac for two years, but is off that now. Since she has been taking herbs and vitamins she can get out of bed more easily in the morning, but she "runs out of steam" by 3 P.M. She is too tired to exercise. These symptoms have increased slowly over the past five years.

The blood test shows nothing greatly out of line. (The 226 cholesterol is not dangerously high, but fits with the research findings that low blood pressure correlates with elevated cholesterol.) Her doctor offered her little except reassurance, "Your blood pressure is so low, you'll live to be a hundred." (See Table 14.1.)

The computer sorts out the data and we begin to see the reasons for the symptoms (see Tables 14.2 and 14.3).

In the left column of Table 14.3 you can see the high alkaline score (anion/cation), which would make it difficult for the minerals to be soluble enough to be useful for her enzyme systems. The hematocrit, hemoglobin, and RBC are high enough to rule out anemia as a cause of fatigue. Note in the far right column more than half the elements are negative, i.e., below the mean; she is nutrient-deficient. Her sodium, calcium, total protein, albumin, iron, GGT (magnesium), and nitrogen elements (BUN, uric acid, creatinine) are all low enough to explain her low blood pressure and fatigue. Nutrients are not getting to her brain to help her think.

The electrolytes (see Table 14.3) are off enough to explain her truncated circulation; she may not be getting enough blood to her brain. The negative values in the liver function reveal where the deficiencies are critical. She needs two therapeutic vitamins a day and three ammonium chloride tablets a day. Eight ounces of two percent milk mixed half and half with the electrolyte solution and drunk twice a day will normalize her calcium.

Within three days of starting the program (see her program checklist, page 171), the blood pressure began to rise, she got her energy back, and her hands and feet began to warm up. In two weeks on the program her blood pressure was a normal 126/85, and she felt well. Her auditory memory is not good, she says, but she has begun to remember some dreams. She likes the smell of B_6. Her depression is lifting.

TABLE 14.1
LABORATORY BLOOD TEST: C.J.

Test	Result		Reference
	In Range	Out of Range	Range
Glucose (Fasting)	89.0		70.0–115.0
Urea Nitrogen	12.0		7.0–25.0
Creatinine	0.9		0.7–1.4
BUN/Creat Ratio	13.3		10.0–24.0
Sodium	140.0		135.0–148.0
Potassium	4.8		3.5–5.3
Chloride	104.0		96.0–112.0
Carbon dioxide	25.0		20.0–34.0
Calcium	9.1		8.5–10.6
Phosphorus, Inorganic	3.6		2.5–4.5
Protein, Total	6.6		6.0–8.5
Albumin	4.2		3.2–5.0
Globulin, Total	2.4		2.2–4.2
A/G Ratio	1.8		0.8–2.0
Bilirubin, Total	0.3		0.2–1.2
Bilirubin, Direct	0.1		0.0–0.3
Bilirubin, Indirect	0.2		0.0–0.9
Alkaline Phosphatase	65.0		20.0–140.0
Lactate Dehydrogenase	134.0		0.0–250.0
GGT	14.0		0.0–45.0
AST (SGOT)	14.0		0.0–50.0
ALT (SGPT)	15.0		0.0–48.0
Uric Acid	4.7		2.5–7.5
Iron, Total	87.0		25.0–170.0
Triglycerides	108.0		20.0–160.0
Cholesterol, Total		226.0 H	<200.0

Complete Blood Count

Test	In Range	Out of Range	Reference Range
White blood cell count	7.1		3.8–10.1
Red blood cell count	4.8		3.9–5.2
Hemoglobin (B)	14.9		12.0–15.6
Hematocrit	44.9		35.0–46.0
MCV	93.6		80.0–100.0
MCH	31.0		27.0–33.0
MCHC	33.1		32.0–36.0
RDW	14.4		9.0–15.0
Platelet count	280.0		130.0–400.0
Platelet count from yellow (ACD) tube			
Neutrophil, SEGS	66.3		40.0–75.0
Lymphocytes	27.0		18.0–47.0
Monocytes	4.5		0.0–12.0
Eosinophils	2.0		0.0–6.0
Basophils	0.2		0.0–2.0

TABLE 14.2
LIFE BALANCES BLOOD TEST EVALUATION

	Result	Low	High	Mean	+ or −	Weighted Deviation
Anion/Cation	15.80	6.00	12.00	9.00	6.80	13.33%
Hematocrit	44.90	35.00	46.00	40.50	4.40	40.00%
Hemoglobin	14.90	12.00	15.60	13.80	1.10	30.56%
Neutrophils	66.30	40.00	75.00	57.50	8.80	25.14%
Potassium	4.80	3.50	5.30	4.40	.40	22.22%
RBC	4.80	3.90	5.20	4.55	.25	19.23%
MCV	93.60	80.00	100.00	90.00	3.60	18.00%
A/G Ratio	1.80	1.00	2.20	1.60	.20	16.67%
MCH	31.00	27.00	33.00	30.00	1.00	16.67%
Triglycerides	108.00	20.00	160.00	90.00	18.00	12.86%
Chloride/CO_2	4.16	3.24	4.75	3.99	.17	11.05%
Chloride	104.00	95.00	110.00	102.50	1.50	10.00%
Cholesterol	226.00	121.00	304.00	212.50	13.50	7.38%
Platelet Est.	280.00	130.00	400.00	265.00	15.00	5.56%
Phosphorus	3.60	2.50	4.50	3.50	.10	5.00%
WBC	7.10	3.80	10.10	6.95	.15	2.38%
LDH	134.00	0.00	270.00	135.00	− 1.00	− .37%
Monocytes	4.50	0.00	10.00	5.00	− .50	− 5.00%
BUN/Creat Ratio	13.30	8.00	20.00	14.00	− .70	− 5.83%
Uric Acid	4.70	2.50	7.50	5.00	− .30	− 6.00%
Albumin	4.20	3.20	5.50	4.35	− .15	− 6.52%
Glucose (Fasting)	89.00	70.00	115.00	92.50	− 3.50	− 7.78%
Globulin	2.40	1.50	3.80	2.65	− .25	− 10.87%
Sodium	140.00	135.00	148.00	141.50	− 1.50	− 11.54%
Alk. Phosphatase	65.00	20.00	140.00	80.00	− 15.00	− 12.50%
Ionized Calcium	4.16	3.80	4.80	4.30	− .14	− 14.11%
CO_2	25.00	20.00	34.00	27.00	− 2.00	− 14.29%
Iron	87.00	40.00	175.00	107.50	− 20.50	− 15.19%
Eosinophils	2.00	0.00	6.00	3.00	− 1.00	− 16.67%
GGT	14.00	0.00	45.00	22.50	− 8.50	− 18.89%
Lymphocytes	27.00	18.00	47.00	32.50	− 5.50	− 18.97%
Creatinine	.90	.70	1.40	1.05	− .15	− 21.43%
Calcium	9.10	8.50	10.60	9.55	− .45	− 21.43%
SGOT	14.00	0.00	50.00	25.00	− 11.00	− 22.00%
BUN	12.00	7.00	25.00	16.00	− 4.00	− 22.22%
MCHC	33.10	32.00	36.00	34.00	− .90	− 22.50%
SGPT	15.00	0.00	55.00	27.50	− 12.50	− 22.73%
Total Protein	6.60	6.00	8.50	7.25	− .65	− 26.00%
Ca/P Ratio	2.53	2.36	3.40	2.88	− .35	− 33.51%
Sodium/Potassium	29.17	27.92	38.57	33.25	− 4.08	− 38.33%
Basophils	.20	0.00	2.00	1.00	− .80	− 40.00%
Total Bilirubin	.30	.20	1.20	.70	− .40	− 40.00%

Avg. Deviation   19.78%

+ or − Deviation   -2.82%

TABLE 14.3
LIFE BALANCES BLOOD TEST EVALUATION: C.J.
Continued

Electrolytes	*Deviation*
Sodium	−11.54%
Potassium	22.22%
Chloride	10.00%
CO_2	−14.29%
Calcium	−21.43%
Total Deviation	15.89%
+ or −	
Deviation	−3.01%

Renal Function	*Deviation*
BUN	−22.22%
Chloride	10.00%
CO_2	−14.29%
Creatinine	−21.43%
Potassium	22.22%
Sodium	−11.54%
Total Deviation	16.95%
+ or −	
Deviation	−6.21%

Liver Function	*Deviation*
SGOT	−22.00%
SGPT	−22.73%
GGT	−18.89%
Total Bilirubin	−40.00%
Alk. Phosphatase	−12.50%
Total Deviation	23.22%
+ or −	
Deviation	−23.22%

Lipids	*Deviation*
Cholesterol	7.38%
Triglycerides	12.86%
Total Deviation	10.12%
+ or −	
Deviation	10.12%

Hematology	*Deviation*
WBC	2.38%
RBC	19.23%
Hemoglobin	30.56%
Hematocrit	40.00%
MCV	18.00%
MCH	16.67%
MCHC	−22.50%
Platelets	5.56%
Total Deviation	19.36%
+ or −	
Deviation	13.74%

Diff. WBC	*Deviation*
Neutrophils	25.14%
Lymphocytes	−18.97%
Monocytes	−5.00%
Eosinophils	−16.67%
Basophils	−40.00%
Total Deviation	21.16%
+ or −	
Deviation	−11.10%

Ratios	*Deviation*
Anion/Cation	113.33%
Ca/P	−33.51%
Na/K	38.33%
Cl/CO_2	11.05%
BUN/Creat	−5.83%
Total Deviation	40.41%
+ or −	
Deviation	9.34%

Proteins	*Deviation*
Total Protein	−26.00%
Albumin	−6.52%
Globulin	−10.87%
A/G Ratio	16.67%
Total Deviation	15.01%
+ or −	
Deviation	−6.68%

LIFE BALANCES, INC.
CHECKLIST

NAME:_____

DATE:_____

BREAKFAST

Take Time
Y/N

☐ [_____] Milk & Electrolytes, 20's, and Multi's
In a 16 ounce glass mix 3 Cap-Fulls green label CONCENTRATE
electrolytes and 16 oz of 2% milk. Take One #20, & TWO Life Balances
TheraVite Multivitamin with the electrolytes and milk.

LUNCH

☐ [_____] Take One #20 with lunch.

DINNER

☐ [_____] Milk & Electrolytes and 20's
In a 16 ounce glass mix 3 Cap-Fulls green label CONCENTRATE
electrolytes and 16 oz of 2% milk. Take One #20 with the electrolytes
and milk.

Special Instructions: Use Salt—Drink Milk
Note: #20 is the ammonium chloride.

* * * * * FILL IN Y (YES), N (NO), & TIME * * * * *

15

The Chemistry of Mental and Emotional Dysfunctions

About ten years ago I was a guest speaker at a church in Ohio. My point was that the body, the mind, and the spirit are all connected one to another, and each has an effect on the others. The minister told me, "In religion we have known for centuries that the body and the mind were connected. It is you doctors who have tried to separate the two." Ever since I studied anatomy I knew that all the parts of the body are connected.

The Busy Brain

When I studied the research in neuroendocrinology, I discovered that the brain has no storage capacity for energy as the liver does. The brain is completely dependent upon the glucose floating in the bloodstream for its energy. The liver and muscles store glycogen ready to be converted to glucose during fasting or exercise. The brain must rely on what is available at any one time.

When God and Mother Nature put mankind together, and decided that newborns would be delivered through the pelvis, they had to make the head small enough to fit through that bony funnel. If the brain was to think great thoughts, they figured, it would have to store glycogen (the body's energy source). But, they reasoned, it would become huge like the liver, and vaginal birth would then be impossible. The compromise was obvious:

No glycogen storage in the brain to energize it; energy must come from the bloodstream.

The brain is the busiest organ we have. Twenty-five percent of the blood from each heartbeat goes to the brain. A child's brain has two to three times the energy needs of the adult. No wonder children flip out when they are stressed on an empty stomach.

The brain also needs nutrients to allow the enzymes to work properly. Take a look at the symptoms that coincide with the various deficiencies in Chapter 6 and notice how many "psycho-neurotic symptoms" there are from fear to fatigue, from anxiety to surliness. They all could be explained by nutrient deficiencies or imbalances.

In my day, if a sick or disturbed patient was not taking hallucinogens, had no fever, or did not have a palpable tumor, he was sent to the psychiatrist. We have since learned that not every emotional glitch is due to our mother's improper rearing techniques. And now, wonder of wonders, psychiatrists are looking into the relationship of emotional problems and their connection with unbalanced neurotransmitters. Psychiatrists and psychologists are learning about the chemistry of emotions. Remember the three Ds of pellagra, a severe vitamin B_3 deficiency: dermatitis, diarrhea, and dementia? Dementia is any symptom from irritability to paranoia—all from a niacin deficiency.

Because I am more skilled at reading the clues in the blood tests, I can often tell what symptoms a client has by looking at the tests without even seeing the client.

ANXIETY

The most common of the "emotional" group of symptoms reported is the feeling of anxiety, the sensation of impending doom. "Something awful is about to happen," is a frequent expression. Anxiety, phobias, and fears are usually experienced by people who are nutrient-deficient: Two-thirds of their test results are below the mean. This is especially true with the GGT, a liver enzyme. The level of this enzyme is dependent upon the body's level of magnesium. Low GGT means low magnesium. High GGT may mean the person is taking too much magnesium, but it could also mean that there *is* something wrong with the liver. (The other liver enzymes are also elevated if the liver is diseased.)

The natural control of anxiety would proscribe sugar, alcohol, caffeine, aspartame. The naturopathic doctor would add the B-complex, calcium, magnesium, tryptophan, bach flowers, and seek to eliminate stress. Herbalists have found the following of great help: *Oxytropis*, *Natrum muriaticum*, *Borax*, *Aluminum*, *Sanic causticum*, *Electrictas*, *Plumbum metallicum*, *Sepia*, *Lilium tigrin*, valerian root, black cohosh, chamomile, hops, skullcap, *Capsicum*, and passion flower.

HYPERACTIVITY

Since most of the hyperactive kids are low in calcium and magnesium, it is easy to see why they are restless, touchy, and distractible. Many have school phobia. I used to believe that hyperactive children only needed to eat more nourishing food. Keeping the blood sugar from fluctuating wildly was my goal. If a child—or adult—has mood swings, like Jekyll and Hyde, it means the blood sugar level is wildly fluctuating. There is no psychiatric condition that makes the mood change so dramatically for no good reason than blood sugar fluctuations. And not from just sugar ingestion, but mood swings may be from eating something allergenic and addicting.

(One mother reported if she asked her seven-year old to take out the garbage, "Like a nice boy," after breakfast, he did it fairly consistently and cheerfully. If, however, she asked him in the same pleasant way *before* his breakfast, he was likely to throw the garbage at her and pull a knife, complaining loudly, "I'm always doing things around here. No way!" She was asking the boy's spinal cord to do a chore that requires the brain's neocortex to be in the neurological [read civilized] loop.)

I advised that these hyper children eat nourishing foods every two to four hours. Albeit inconvenient, this prevented the swings of attention, temperament, and attitude. Why doesn't everyone have these problems? I assumed it was genetics, the great wastebasket of explanations. Most of these came from families where alcoholism, diabetes, obesity, or hyperactivity—all sugar-related problems—lived. I felt that if we could just feed everyone in the world some nourishing food every two to four hours, hyperactivity, crime, and depression would disappear from the face of the earth. Graze.

Well, it does work, but not on everyone. Hypoglycemia, however, is a valid explanation for those with depression, especially if there is no good reason for the sadness. We know now that the type and amounts of food, sugar, aspartame, vitamins, minerals, toxic products, and amino acids are responsible for thoughts, feelings, and behavior. Herbalists have used valerian, passiflora, and hops with some success.

A Child with Hyperactivity

I used to think that I had most of the answers to the all too common hyperactive child, now called Attention Deficit Disability (ADA). I asked the parents to stop the child from eating anything he/she wanted, including sugar and milk, and put the child on calcium (1,000 mg) and magnesium (500 mg) daily. It did work, but not on every one I treated; my figures were that about 80 percent were 60 to 100 percent better. But I was guessing.

Here follows the not unusual story of a little girl, S.S., age six years. Four feet; fifty-two pounds. The mother says she has always been a difficult child. She had no ear infections as an infant, but did start to hold her breath at twelve months of age when angry or frustrated. She turned blue and had a seizure with a stiffening of her body and the eyes rolling up. Very frightening. She always seemed tense; she had hard muscles. She ran on her tiptoes. She had trouble relaxing and going to sleep. She had ups and downs of mood and activity, and her attention span was always short. Somehow the mother and daughter survived. The teacher in school finally realized that S.S. was somewhat hyper and something must be done. The mother put her on calcium and magnesium, but it was not much help. She started the Life Balances program in April 1993, but because it was slow the mother tried Ritalin. With that S.S. really went wild and crazy. A chiropractor noted that she had allergies and hypoglycemia. She does better if she eats every two hours, especially during school.

Here are the blood tests as sorted out by the Life Balances computer program (see Tables 15.1 and 15.2). Note the high anion/cation score; she is very alkaline. This is probably the reason the calcium and magnesium were not very effective earlier; they were not soluble in her alkaline body. The high eosinophil count corroborates the allergy theory, but could also mean parasites. The low value for serum iron suggests one possible

TABLE 15.1
LIFE BALANCES BLOOD TEST EVALUATION: S.S.

	Result	Low	High	Mean	+ or −	Weighted Deviation
Anion/Cation	17.30	6.00	12.00	9.00	8.30	138.33%
Eosinophils	7.10	1.00	5.00	3.00	4.10	102.50%
Triglycerides	134.00	10.00	120.00	65.00	69.00	62.73%
Chloride/CO$_2$	4.77	3.86	4.75	4.30	.47	52.55%
BUN/Creat Ratio	23.80	10.00	24.00	17.00	6.80	48.57%
Lymphocytes	57.10	30.00	60.00	45.00	12.10	40.33%
BUN	19.00	8.00	21.00	14.50	4.50	34.62%
LDH	196.00	0.00	250.00	125.00	71.00	28.40%
Chloride	105.00	95.00	108.00	101.50	3.50	26.92%
Creatinine	.80	.30	1.00	.65	.15	21.43%
Phosphorus	5.00	3.00	6.00	4.50	.50	16.67%
MCHC	34.50	32.00	36.00	34.00	.50	12.50%
Monocytes	5.60	2.00	8.00	5.00	.60	10.00%
Glucose (Fasting)	89.00	60.00	110.00	85.00	4.00	8.00%
MCH	27.20	24.00	30.00	27.00	.20	3.33%
Calcium	9.60	8.50	10.60	9.55	.05	2.38%
Ionized Calcium	4.32	3.80	4.80	4.30	.02	2.31%
Albumin	4.40	3.20	5.50	4.35	.05	2.17%
Alk. Phosphatase	246.00	60.00	417.00	238.50	7.50	2.10%
Total Protein	6.80	5.50	8.00	6.75	.05	2.00%
Sodium/Potassium	32.56	26.36	38.57	32.47	.09	.74%
Hemoglobin	12.50	11.50	13.50	12.50	0.00	0.00%
RBC	4.60	3.90	5.30	4.60	0.00	0.00%
Sodium	140.00	135.00	145.00	140.00	0.00	0.00%
Platelet Est.	264.00	130.00	400.00	265.00	−1.00	−.37%
Globulin	2.40	1.40	3.50	2.45	−.05	−2.38%
A/G Ratio	1.80	1.00	2.70	1.85	−.05	−2.94%
SGOT	23.00	0.00	50.00	25.00	−2.00	−4.00%
Potassium	4.30	3.50	5.50	4.50	−.20	−10.00%
Hematocrit	36.30	34.00	40.00	37.00	−.70	−11.67%
Neutrophils	29.90	17.00	53.00	35.00	−5.10	−14.17%
Cholesterol	184.00	121.00	304.00	212.50	−28.50	−15.57%
MCV	78.70	75.00	87.00	81.00	−2.30	−19.17%
CO$_2$	22.00	20.00	28.00	24.00	−2.00	−25.00%
SGPT	10.00	0.00	45.00	22.50	−12.50	−27.78%
GGT	13.00	0.00	65.00	32.50	−19.50	−30.00%
Uric Acid	3.40	2.50	7.50	5.00	−1.60	−32.00%
Iron	59.00	35.00	175.00	105.00	−46.00	−32.86%
Ca/P Ratio	1.92	1.77	2.83	2.30	−.38	−35.63%
Total Bilirubin	.30	.20	1.20	.70	−.40	−40.00%
WBC	4.60	5.00	16.00	10.50	−5.90	−53.64%
Basophils	.30	1.00	2.00	1.50	−1.20	−120.00%

Avg. Deviation   26.09%

+ or − Deviation   3.37%

TABLE 15.2
LIFE BALANCES BLOOD TEST EVALUATION: S.S.
Continued

Electrolytes	Deviation
Sodium	0.00%
Potassium	10.00%
Chloride	26.92%
CO_2	−25.00%
Calcium	2.38%
Total Deviation	12.86%
+ or − Deviation	−1.14%

Renal Function	Deviation
BUN	34.62%
Chloride	26.92%
CO_2	−25.00%
Creatinine	21.43%
Potassium	−10.00%
Sodium	0.00%
Total Deviation	19.66%
+ or − Deviation	7.99%

Liver Function	Deviation
SGOT	−4.00%
SGPT	−27.78%
GGT	−30.00%
Total Bilirubin	−40.00%
Alk. Phosphatase	2.10%
Total Deviation	20.78%
+ or − Deviation	−19.94%

Lipids	Deviation
Cholesterol	−15.57%
Triglycerides	62.73%
Total Deviation	39.15%
+ or − Deviation	23.58%

Hematology	Deviation
WBC	−53.64%
RBC	0.00%
Hemoglobin	0.00%
Hematocrit	−11.67%
MCV	−19.17%
MCH	3.33%
MCHC	12.50%
Platelets	−.37%
Total Deviation	12.58%
+ or − Deviation	−8.63%

Diff. WBC	Deviation
Neutrophils	−14.17%
Lymphocytes	40.33%
Monocytes	10.00%
Eosinophils	102.50%
Basophils	−120.00%
Total Deviation	57.40%
+ or − Deviation	3.73%

Ratios	Deviation
Anion/Cation	138.33%
Ca/P	−35.63%
Na/K	.74%
Cl/CO_2	52.55%
BUN/Creat	48.57%
Total Deviation	55.16%
+ or − Deviation	40.91%

Proteins	Deviation
Total Protein	2.00%
Albumin	2.17%
Globulin	−2.38%
A/G Ratio	−2.94%
Total Deviation	2.37%
+ or − Deviation	−.29%

LIFE BALANCES, INC.
CHECKLIST

NAME: S.S.

DATE: Apr 30, 1993

BREAKFAST

Take   Time
Y/N

☐ ☐ Milk & Electrolytes, 13's, 20's, and Multi's
In a 8 ounce glass mix 4 oz green label electrolytes and 4 oz of 2% milk.
Take Four #13's, One #20, & One Life Balances TheraVite Multivitamin
with the electrolytes and milk. On Mondays, Wednesdays, & Fridays
Take One #16.

NOON
☐ ☐ 13's and 15's
Take Four #13's & One #15 with Lunch.

DINNER
☐ ☐ Milk & Electrolytes, 13's, and 20's
In a 8 ounce glass mix 4 oz green label electrolytes and 4 oz of 2% milk.
Take Four #13 & One #20 with electrolytes and milk.

BEDTIME
☐ ☐ 13's
Take Four #13's with a Snack.

Special Instructions: After 1 week delete the #15's & #20's
Note: #13 is betaine HCl, #20 is ammonium chloride, #16 is
magnesium.

* * * * * FILL IN Y (YES), N (NO), & TIME * * * * *

reason for inappropriate cerebral function, although she is not anemic. Serum iron helps to nou rish the brain. The high phosphorus and normal calcium throws off the CA/P ratio, which has much to do with cell function. The GGT (magnesium) is very low and that helps to explain the breath-holding seizures, the poor attention span, and her distractibility. (She is very ticklish.) The second page of the evaluation (Table 15.2) shows the poor liver function and the distorted ratios. The recommendations: electrolytes mixed with 2 percent milk, betaine hydrochloride, ammonium chloride (acidifiers), a multivitamin each day, and a magnesium tablet three times a week (see Life Balances Checklist, page 179).

Another blood test will be done to see the progress and make necessary changes. I thought it important to add B_6, 100 mg daily, because she has trouble with dream recall. It should help, but the bottle of B_6 should smell good, too.

NEUROTRANSMITTERS

Since 1950 when Dr. Abram Hoffer clearly showed that niacin deficiency explained some forms of schizophrenia, doctors have been busy proving (and trying to disprove) his original observations. Although schizophrenia has a basis in genetics, he believed that "chromosomes and genes cannot by themselves cause anything. It it the combination of genes and their chemical cellular environment that determines the final outcome. The genes have special requirements. If these are met, no disease will result."

It is abundantly clear that foods alter moods, thoughts, and perceptions. Certain foods change the concentrations of neurotransmitters (NT) that, in turn change mood, garble thoughts, and distort perceptions. If carbohydrates are eaten at bedtime, the insulin produced lowers the blood sugar, but also pushes the small chain amino acids into storage. This reduces the competition of the amino acids through the blood-brain barrier, allowing tryptophan, a large molecule, to have priority. Once into the brain circulation, it produces serotonin, which has a calming effect on the nervous system, and, of course, helps the insomniacal patient relax and sleep.

Neurotransmitter synthesis and release are the result of changes in the availability of precursors from the blood plasma. Sensors have the potential for providing the brain with information about the body's metabolic states. The brain then will initiate foraging activities to search for the foods that contain the specific nutrients that will induce sleep, alertness, or whatever.

It has been found that the neurotransmitter levels in blood platelets correlate positively with the levels of NTs in the brain. The metabolites of these NTs can be measured in the urine. Here are a few of the precursors, their regulating cofactors, and the NTs they produce:

TABLE 15.3
CREATING NEUROTRANSMITTERS

Precursor	Regulating Cofactors	Neurotransmitter
Serine, choline	Coenzyme A, choline	Acetylcholine
Histidine, histamine	Cu, Zn, Mn, B_6	Imidazole
Tyrosine, tyramine	Cu, Mg, B_3, B_6, AA, FA	Epinephrine
Phenylalanine	Cu, Mg, B_3, B_6, AA, FA	Norepinephrine
Phenylalanine	Fe, B_3, Biotin	Dopamine
Tryptophan	FA, B_3, B_6	Serotonin
Glutamate	B_6, Biotin	Gamma-amino butyrate

A cursory glance at this table gives some insight why a hyper child might be calmed with magnesium and B_6; they are helping him make his own norepinephrine so his limbic system can filter out the distractions coming into his brain through his eyes and ears.

The measurements of the NT will reveal deficiencies or excesses. These measurements can be correlated with behavior or psychiatric dysfunctions. The cofactors responsible for the activation of the regulating enzymes tend to increase the production of the deficient NT. These are the amino acids, the minerals, and the vitamins. Remember the chemical rule: The greater the concentration, the more rapid the reaction. Because of individual biochemistry, some people cannot manufacture enough of NTs to keep them from anxiety, depression, or psychosis.

NT PRECURSORS

Genetic tendencies do not have to appear unless the lifestyle and the diet are faulty. If any of the regulatory factors are *deficient* in the diet, or if a person has a genetic *dependency* on any of them, the individual elements smell good and should be taken. The most commonly needed ones are magnesium, B_3 (niacin), B_6 (pyridoxine), iron, and folic acid. The minerals that come in the dropper bottles help to fulfill the precursor needs of the enzymes so they are able to make the neurotransmitters. This method does take longer to control unacceptable behavior and thoughts than a prescription for tranquilizers, antidepressants, or antipsychotic drugs, but is certainly safer and more accurate because one is taking the specific missing elements necessary to make the NTs. Some nutritionally oriented psychiatrists use drugs temporarily while awaiting the vitamins, minerals, and amino acids to manufacture the NTs naturally.

Some dietary precursors of the NTs: Lecithin from eggs and soy provide choline in a form that rides through the blood-brain barrier to increase the acetylcholine and improve memory. Tyramine from cheddar and similar cheeses is metabolized to norepinephrine. Histidine from protein becomes histamine. Tyrosine from wheat germ and fowl allows the easy manufacture of epinephrine, norepinephrine, and dopamine. Glutamine comes from wild game, granola, and ricotta cheese. And sulfur amino acids are derived from yogurt and duck—important for methylation reactions.

Many people, however, have digestion problems and cannot break down the protein foods they eat to these important amino acids. These freeform amino acids may be necessary for those with a malabsorption problems.

SCHIZOPHRENIA

Russell Jaffe, MD, Ph.D. and Oscar Kruesi, M.D., have outlined the biochemical needs of various psychotic illnesses and how to evaluate them "(The Biochemical-Immunology Window: A Molecular View of Psychiatric Case Management" *Journal of Applied Nutrition*, 44: #2, 1992). They followed the lead of the late Dr. Carl Pfeiffer who found the following types of schizophrenia and their basic characteristics:

Low Histamine Type (40 percent of schizophrenics) do better if they have the following supplements: beta-carotene, vitamin C,

B-complex, extra folate and B_{12}, histidine, quercetin, GLA fatty acid, iron, zinc, molybdenum, manganese. These people sometimes can be relied upon to tell which supplements are best for them. Vitamin C, niacin, folic acid would probably smell good to them. When they take the niacin, they usually do not develop that uncomfortable histamine flush, because they have so little histamine in their system.

High Histamine Type (15 percent of schizophrenics) usually has an allergic history with hives, asthma, and eczema. Hypertension and migraines are also common. They respond to methionine, zinc, manganese, molybdenum, vitamin C, and essential fatty acids.

Pyrroluric Type (15 percent of schizophrenics) show the mauve factor in the urine. They may respond to zinc, B_6, and manganese.

Nutrient Deficient Type (15 percent of schizophrenics) usually have a history of allergies, mood swings, and digestive disorders. Blood tests reveal some or many of their vitamin and mineral deficiencies. They may show many of the symptoms and signs suggested in Chapter 6. This group of mentally disturbed patients, especially, are able to tell their needs by the smelling and tasting tests. Many from this group are prone to heavy metal toxicities. Hair tests are efficient at revealing the metal and the amount of the load.

Immunoreactive Type (15 percent of schizophrenics) are those who react to foods and chemicals. Gluten sensitivity is an example. Milk lactalbumin is one of the most common food sensitivities that could make one classified as psychotic. Some doctors who test for food sensitivities have found that 80 percent of those who hear voices have positive food tests. When the offenders (milk, coffee, corn, soy, wheat, eggs, nuts, etc.) are eliminated, the voices cease. Many of these foods cause atrophy of the intestinal lining and the vitamins and minerals in the swallowed but undigested food are not absorbed. Most of these people need digestive enzymes, and the betaine might even smell good to them. They show nutrient deficiencies on the blood tests and the magnesium and potassium is very low, aggravating their mental symptoms. The authors are careful to point out that these various types commonly overlap. "Nutrient deficient and immunologic types overlap with more than half of all schizophrenic and mood-disordered patients we evaluate."

They also are aware of the bilateral direction of interactions between the central nervous system and the immune system. The new term psychoneuroimmunology fits with everything we are now learning about "mind over matter." There is a food-mood connection!

The treatment of nervous and mental disorders has been rife with therapeutic guesswork. Now thanks to the Life Balances program and the work of researchers such as Dr. Jaffe, we are able to provide more specific nutrients to the treatment of these "mysterious" diseases, and offer more than just hope and luck.

Naturopathic physicians have had some success with homeopathy, bach flowers, *Aesculus hippocastanum*, *Medicago sativa*, and ginkgo.

Aggressive Behavior

Allopathic control consists of incarceration, behavior modification, and psychiatry. Doctors who try a more natural control would search for heavy metal poisonings (the hair test is valuable for these metals), especially copper, lead, and cadmium. Bach flowers, homeopathy, and eliminating food allergies are worthwhile pursuits. Dr. William Walsh, Ph.D., found that violent criminals had high levels of lead, cadmium, iron, and calcium, and lower levels of zinc in their hair than normal people.

Alzheimer's Disease

The allopathic control offers little as no one yet knows the cause of the problem. It was once called presenile psychosis as it appeared in some people under sixty years of age. Small strokes, and cerebral atrophy can be ruled out by tests. Doctors who follow the course of these people have found that aluminum seems to be lodged in the brain in critical areas. Some have found that large doses of B_{12} and folic acid by injection have been helpful. Vitamin C has been of some benefit to help purge the aluminum or heavy metals stored in the brain. Life Balances has discovered that as we age we become more alkaline, and the aluminum molecule becomes smaller and can more easily move from the circulation into the brain. Zinc seems to be helpful in controlling the aluminum.

Central Nervous System Damage

My friend and Life Balances supporter, Patricia Kane, Ph.D., has graciously offered me the use of the following histories of children with central nervous system damage.

Emily was born in January 1988, after an eight-month pregnancy during which her mother consumed enormous amounts of aspartame. She was placed on a Similac formula. She showed normal development and was walking at fifteen months of age. But from that point on she deteriorated. She lost her gross and fine motor skills. By 1993, at age five years when Dr. Kane saw her, she had lost her ability to walk or even crawl. She could not pick up objects, was unable to feed herself, and was only able to whisper as she was too weak to speak. She had received osteopathic treatment, but with little benefit. Her IQ was 113. Her diet had been a sugar cereal for breakfast, the public school lunch, and snacks of cookies and potato chips. Dinner was a hot dog, pork or beef, corn, broccoli, white rice, or noodles. She craved cheese, butter, chocolate, and pizza. She drank soft drinks with aspartame, and little water. She disliked orange juice. Margarine and hydrogenated fats were always present in her diet. No supplements have ever been given.

When Dr. Kane saw her in May of 1993, she was very weak. Thirty-nine pounds, 49 inches, T = 98.2, pulse = 66, and blood pressure 80/50. No amalgam fillings. Fingers long and thin. She had some white spots on her nails. When lying supine she could pull her body to the left, but could not pull her legs to the left, so she became distraught. She was unable to hold her head erect for more than a few seconds, she was so weak. She was uncomfortable with sounds. She demanded constant attention. She was sensitive to sugar, wheat, chocolate, and oranges. Her blood chemistry showed dysfunction in the nitrogen-bearing components, high sodium, electrolyte imbalance, high calcium level, elevated triglycerides, alkalinity, and nutrient density. She had 1s on the smelling test scores for B_1, B_6, B_{12}, folic acid, PABA, calcium, and ammonium chloride, but all the rest were 9s or 10s to her.

Her diet was changed to simple, wholesome foods and the elimination of hydrogenated fats, sugar, chemicals, wheat, chocolate, and orange. She drank the electrolyte solution, vinegar water, the trace mineral drink, folic acid, B_6, B_1, bioflavonoids, coenzyme Q_{10}, ammonium chloride, octacosanol (dry form), and B_{12}.

Within two weeks she was stronger as evidenced by her increased activity level, she was talking above a whisper, participating in the school activities, seemed happier, whined less, could pick up and manipulate objects, and was able to move on her own. Her parents and teachers were overjoyed. Her use of nutrients was determined by her sense of smell and taste. Dr. Kane added essential fatty acid nutrients, previously missing from her prior impoverished diet.

Dr. Kane's research discovered a link between Emily's symptoms and her exposure to aspartame *in utero*. Dr. Kane contacted Dr. Woodrow C. Monte, Ph.D., R.D., who had written a paper a decade ago entitled "Aspartame: Methanol and the Public Health." His investigation suggested that the methanol in aspartame may be dehydrogenated by fermentation into formaldehyde (embalming fluid) and attach itself to protein. It can thus destroy the myelin around the nerve cells. Rebuilding this myelin seemed logical and specific to the condition of this little girl. The electrolytes were important to carry the fatty acids into her body and brain.

In another month Emily was walking and talking. A new MRI test showed increase in the white matter of the nervous system.

AYLA, THE MIRACLE BABY

What would you do if you gave birth to a 700-gram baby after only five months of gestation? Turn your back and give her up? It would seem sensible given the long expensive road—if she survives—to retardation, blindness, spasticity, or at least extreme hyperactivity.

Ayla happened to be born in a hospital where life-support systems were available, but this tiny little girl kept slipping to the edge of death despite the machinery; but she could always be revived. Ayla, to her mother, was becoming a "factor" to be reckoned with. She was a fighter. Her mother, Mrs. V., became involved. She watched, monitored, and asked questions. She said prayers. She talked to Ayla.

Ayla was fed intravenously with water, glucose, and electrolytes. After a month of borderline survival, breast milk was added by an oral tube. Then folic acid and vitamin E were added. Her heart and lungs "forgot" to function every once in a while, but after a few weeks of constant vigilance with the mother and the monitoring machines, her condition stabilized. Dr. Kane was asked to "take a look." Dr. Kane knew from personal experience that the nervous system needs a great deal of nourishment—more than just water, minerals, and glucose.

Blood chemistry studies were limited but did reveal nutrient deficiencies. (The lack of many essential nutrients suggested the reason for the early delivery.) Dr. Kane realized the mother's feeble vegetarian diet was not sufficient for her own body, much less her breast milk. Kane outlined a nutrient-dense diet for Mrs. V., including some fish, eggs, seeds, nuts, legumes, and of course, vegetables. Essential fatty acids were added to the mother's diet (flax, evening primrose oil, wheat germ oil, and salmon oil). The baby also received color, sound, and aromatherapy.

When Ayla was about four pounds, she was moved out of the ICU and placed in the regular nursery, and was soon released from the hospital—with monitoring wires attached! Analysis of her blood showed alkalinity, low hemoglobin, low nitrogen elements, lack of ionized calcium—in general, low mineral density. A mixture of liver, organic meats, and pulverized bone was put down the tube. Her formula at that time was ⅓ breast milk, ⅓ soy formula, and ⅓ electrolyte solution. She also got the liquid vitamin and mineral drops. The mother and Dr. Kane found that if she were fed sitting upright, she could swallow more easily. She was fed every two hours.

Dr. Kane described her one-year-old birthday party last spring. ". . . a party of balloons, streamers, natural carrot cake and Rice Dream ice cream. Her enjoyment was evident as she smashed her cake into the carpet and bonked another baby on the head with her horn-blower and cheered as we sang happy birthday." A survivor. A miracle baby. You cannot make a body without the proper nutrients.

MARY OF THE LIGHT

In the fall of 1992, Mary, a nine-month-old normal baby choked on a bit of walnut in her banana nut cake. Slapping her chest, using the Heimlich maneuver, turning her upside down, and trying to finger the piece from her throat were all unsuccessful. The baby was blue and limp when the mother got her to the closest emergency room twenty-five minutes later. Using instruments in the ER further damaged her throat and lungs, but at least an airway was established and she was connected to a respirator.

In the ambulance to another hospital the tank ran out of oxygen (!) so for another seventeen minutes she was deprived of oxygen. Cardiac arrest and coma followed. She was quickly hooked up to oxygen and a respirator, which saved her tenuous life despite one collapsed lung and blood in both lungs. It took four days to get the oxygen saturation in her blood close to normal. Pneumonia was the next insult. She was finally ready for release in a few weeks, but what a change from that fateful day. A CAT scan revealed extensive brain damage. She had to be tube-fed, her eyes rolled upward most of the time, and because she could not swallow, her saliva had to be suctioned every few minutes, and she was fed by a naso-gastric tube.

Mary's mother was told by all the medical personnel who dealt with this crippled, spastic, nonresponsive child that she should be institutionalized as she was a "just a vegetable." Undaunted, the mother tried a number of approaches. The Doman–Delacato method of patterning was frustrating because Mary's rigidity precluded all but a slight response; but she kept at it. Then Mary's mother asked Dr. Kane to try her methods. When Dr. Kane first saw Mary in early 1993 (age one year) she was shocked: "Mary's body was rigid, her back and hips twisted, her skin pale, her tiny legs were like two thin, straight sticks, and she was severely underweight. Her face was in a grimace. It was as if Mary were locked in time, waiting for someone to help her through her nightmare . . ." Kane began.

Her blood chemistries revealed low-nutrient density and a high state of alkalinity. Part of the problem was the small size of the N–G tube and the fact that all food had to be liquefied. Here is what Dr. Kane had her take daily: 1) Milk, electrolyte solution, egg, maple syrup; 2) liquefied organic vegetables, liver, black beans, vitamins, minerals, and electrolytes; 3) organic fruit juice, liquid minerals; 4) strained potatoes, turkey or chicken, almond butter, vitamins, minerals, electrolytes, and essential fatty acids. Vinegar water was also given between feedings to help control the alkalinity.

In two weeks Mary gained two pounds and lost 85 percent of her rigidity. She slept longer and more comfortably, needed less suctioning, her rashes cleared, and her bowel movements became normal. Stimulation to her sense organs and her brain were done with colors, sounds, and aromas. Various textures were placed next to her skin to stimulate the sense of touch. Patterning was obviously easier to perform and seemed to be helping.

By measuring her temperature, pulse, and blood pressure, Kane was able to determine the amounts of fluid and electrolytes Mary needed. Family, friends, and therapists were all involved in Mary's care: patterning, talking, hugging. Dr. Kane used every therapy she knew to help this little girl along with the Life Balances program: craniosacral, the Beck Brain Tuner, electro-accupressure, massage, Trager movements.

By May 1993, Mary had gained six pounds, grown two inches, could sit alone for two minutes, and had color in her cheeks. She could follow simple commands. Mary's full name in Spanish is Maria De La Luz, or Mary of the light. Mary's story shows that there is hope for these hopeless children.

Depression

The allopathic control is pretty much limited to the antidepressants and lithium, if the depression is the cyclic type. Psychotherapy appears to be only adjunctive. If the depression arrives in November and disappears in May, it is assumed to be the Seasonally Adjusted Depression (SAD) and is treated with lights. Many doctors who practice natural methods of care find that hypoglycemia is the first condition to address, especially if the depression comes and goes. They, of course, stop the aspartame, and try biotin, folic acid, B_6, B_2, B_{12}, C, magnesium, calcium, tryptophan, phenylalanine, homeopathy, bach flowers, *Pulsatilla*, *Caulophylum thalicroides*, *Passiflora incarnata*, *Hypericum*.

Dizziness

Middle ear problems must be ruled out. Some of these people are having transient ischemic attacks, and epilepsy may be masking as dizziness. Anemia will make people dizzy, as well as low blood sugar, and low blood pressure. Low thyroid function would show some other signs of its presence. Pantothenic acid has been helpful for some.

Epilepsy

Epilepsy is a frightening disorder. It is a loss of consciousness for seconds or minutes and is usually accompanied by involuntary muscle spasms, localized or generalized. Seizures are a good example of how the chemistry of the body can affect the nervous system in a dramatic way. Apparently there is a deficiency in the activity of the sodium/potassium adenosine-triphosphatase-membrane pump in the tiny area on the neuron where the seizure begins. It is called an "irritable focus." Drug control to soothe the excitability of this focus is a disappointing 50 to 70 percent and is often associated with uncomfortable side effects, mainly drowsiness.

In normal nerve fiber function a wave of depolarization travels down the axon (nerve fiber) until it gets to the end where its unique neurotransmitter is released, which stimulates the next nerve or a gland. At that spot of depolarization sodium rushes in and the potassium flows out; the nerve fiber then has the same charge on the inside of the cell membrane as on the outside. Then this ATPase pump moves the sodium out and the potassium in to reestablish the polarity—like a recharged battery.

Injuries, infections, tumors, vascular accidents, and congenital malformations are the time-honored causes usually listed. In the last few decades, however, nutrient excesses and deficiencies have proven to be inciting agents to seizures. Hypoglycemia (90 percent of people with seizures have periodic or low blood sugar) has been known to be a factor since 1934. "Electrolyte balance is disturbed and there is a tendency to alkalosis" (Natelson, et al., *Clinical Chemistry*, 25 (6), 1979, pp. 889–897). There is a high percentage of subnormal glucose tolerance tests in epilepsy (Mackay, E.W.J. and Barbash, H., *Journal of Mental Science*, 72:83–85, 1931).

Magnesium deficiency is especially common in epileptics. Tetany and convulsions were first shown to occur in magnesium-deficient rats in 1932. A small but significantly lower level of serum magnesium in epileptic outpatients was observed in 1976 (Christiansen et al). Epileptic convulsions in a physically well-trained man occurred after four hours of continuous exercise in hot conditions. Low-serum magnesium was the only biochemical parameter. (*Aviation Space and Environmental Medicine*, July 1979, pp. 734–5.) Symptoms of magnesium deficiency include muscle tremors and convulsive seizures. In one trial of thirty epileptic patients, 450 mg of magnesium daily successfully controlled seizures in all thirty patients. (Pfeiffer, Carl, *Mental and Elemental Nutrients*, p. 278.) Low-serum magnesium is associated with convulsions in 22 percent, hallucinations in 44 percent, mental confusion in 78 percent, disorientation in 83 percent, and 100 percent of those with low magnesium were easily startled. The normal functions of the nerve fibers are influenced by the concentration and the ratios of the calcium and the magnesium; these minerals control the speed of ingress and egress of the sodium and potassium at the nerve cell wall.

Epileptic patients had significantly lower selenium levels than any group except those with cancer. (*Bulletin of Environmental Contamination and Toxicology:* 26, (4) 1981, pp. 400–471.) Manganese may be low in those with epilepsy. Serum copper, lead, mercury may be high in those with epilepsy. Folic acid, vitamin D, taurine, and B_6 may help control convulsions. The neurotransmitter GABA has a calming or inhibitory effect on the nervous system. B_6 is necessary for the synthesis of GABA.

Homeopathy can control epilepsy. Check for parasites. Herbs that can be helpful include indigo, *Atropa belladonna*, *Pulsatilla*, *Magnesia phosphorica*, and chlorophyll.

A BOY WITH SEIZURES

J.D. is a six-year-old boy who had seizures several times a day since he was an infant. The susceptibility to seizures may have been due to the formaldehyde outgassing (evaporating) from the new trailer in which he and his family were living. His first seizure occurred at age eight months and was felt to be triggered by the odor of the kerosene lantern burning in that trailer. The family moved out of the trailer when he was about eighteen months old and the seizures slowed down. They began again with renewed vigor after he had eaten a pesticide-laced watermelon at age three years.

Drugs for seizure control were largely ineffective. To stop the seizures completely, a dose had to be given that made him semicomatose. The laboratory tests showed that he was moderately alkaline, his calcium level was below the mean, the GGT (a clue about magnesium deficiency) was down, and the BUN, creatinine, and uric acid were well below the mean, as were most of the blood results; he was nutrient-deficient. He was given milk mixed with electrolyte solution, ammonium chloride, iron, and the mineral drops mixed with fruit juice. On the Life Balances program, he slowly responded with fewer seizures, but was never seizure-free. The alkalosis seems to make his nervous system overly excitable, as the minerals are less soluble in an alkaline medium. Vinegar mixed with water was very helpful.

EPILEPSY IN AN ADULT

D.V. is about sixty years old and a fighter. "I have had epilepsy for forty-five years. I spent thirteen years of my childhood in a hospital with no success for treatment using drugs. I managed to lead as normal a life as possible and in spite of the seizures, I did achieve all my goals." In 1982 after eight years as a legal secretary for the Justice Department her superiors wanted to retire her on disability. Her condition was getting worse despite trying all the new drugs that were being synthesized. She resigned from her job, took her retirement funds, which lasted about a year, and threw all her drugs down the toilet. She read about nutrition. For the past ten years besides these seizures she suffered from migraine headaches, enough to incapacitate her; anemia, nausea, and hypoglycemia. Get this: "I was turned down by Social Security because I was not taking drugs, even though I took drugs for forty-six years with thirteen years in a hospital and no success."

In 1982 she started on a nutrition program and the seizures were reduced from twelve per month down to four. The side effects from the drugs also disappeared.

Her blood test last year showed that she was alkaline and we suggested that she drink an eight-ounce glass of water containing a teaspoon of vinegar twice a day because her sodium was elevated and the blood test showed that she was alkaline.

A recent letter: "I have been taking the vinegar for six days and the vitamins and, believe it or not, after forty-six years of symptoms and seizures, the symptoms faded the first day I took the vinegar and the water. I guess it is a dream come true. This will become the answer to most of our health problems, and could very well correct the problems we face in crime and violence through our nation." Now she can go back to working as a temporary typist.

Fatigue

Allopathic doctors would first try to find some chronic infection, such as tuberculosis, mononucleosis, or hypothyroid function to explain it. Blood tests would reveal some evidence of a disease. Anemia would be a prime suspect. If nothing is found they would search for stressors in the patient's life, and then prescribe some antidepressant, or even Ritalin. Doctors using more natural control would first change the diet and proscribe sugar, alcohol, and junk food. Fresh fruits and vegetables would be the main diet. Food sensitivities would be searched for. If the temperature is low, they might place the patient on thyroid. The following herbs are useful: Gingko, ephedra, ginseng, gotu kola, cayenne, acacia, and guarana. Bee pollen, C, E, GH_3, octacosanol, brewer's yeast, desiccated liver have all been found useful.

Here is the story of a lady with Chronic Fatigue Syndrome:

CHRONIC FATIGUE SYNDROME

There are perhaps a score of diseases that fit under the name of CFS. To a certain extent, the Life Balances program does not need to know the name of the disease. It only needs to know that there are chemical deviations from the mean, sets out to correct them, and the malady should take care of itself. It is difficult for the program to factor in such immutables as a stressful job or living with surly in-laws.

P. W. is a thirty-two-year-old woman, 5 feet 11 inches, 143 pounds, who, with her husband, runs a restaurant in western

Kentucky. For the last two years, she has suffered from repeated infections every six to nine weeks. These are manifested by low grade fever, sore throat, and a persistent cough and extreme fatigue. Chiropractic treatments and antibiotics have not lifted her fatigue nor prevented the recurrences of the illness. Each attack has been more severe and has lasted longer. "I have no immunity."

Here is the blood work right from the laboratory (see Table 15.4). Every test is within the lab's "normal" range so the casual, medically trained health provider might say, "Your exam and the blood tests are all normal. Would you like some Valium? How about taking some antibiotic daily for a year or two to prevent the recurrences? Are you having some stress? How about a psychiatrist?"

What a difference in the perception of her lab work once the results have been run through the Life Balances computer data analysis (see Tables 15.5 and 15.6).

First scan the left-hand column. The BUN/creatinine ratio is out of line. The next item is the anion/cation, indicating that she is slightly alkaline. The neutrophils are up slightly due to the recent infection, but the hematocrit, the red blood cell count, and the hemoglobin are right up there; she is not anemic. Now drop your gaze to the bottom of that first column and you will see her deficiencies: The uric acid and creatinine are very low, meaning that she is not getting nitrogen. We don't usually see a level of sodium so low as this; sodium is necessary to help the body fight infection. It may not be good to have a cholesterol so low; it is necessary to act as an antioxidant. The GGT is a clue about the level of magnesium; magnesium is needed in a hundred or more enzyme systems. Calcium and ionized calcium, along with sodium, help protect the cell walls from the invasion of infection. The albumin is needed to make antibodies; it is a little low.

Look at the last column. About 60 percent of her values are in the negative range. That means that she is nutrient deficient. Her body needs some rebuilding.

This reveals rather clearly that she needs some nutritional help, especially in the liver enzymes. The Life Balances's chemist put her on the electrolyte solution mixed with 2 percent milk (sixteen ounces twice a day), ammonium chloride twice a day to provide extra nitrogen and control the alkalinity, and one therapeutic, all-purpose vitamin a day, and a magnesium tablet

TABLE 15.4
LABORATORY BLOOD TEST: P.W.

Report Status Final Test	Result		Reference
	In Range	Out of Range	Range
Glucose (Fasting)	85.0		70.0–115.0
Urea Nitrogen	15.0		7.0–25.0
Creatinine	0.8		0.7–1.4
BUN/Creat Ratio	18.8		10.0–24.0
Sodium	137.0		135.0–148.0
Potassium	4.5		3.5–5.3
Chloride	103.0		96.0–112.0
Carbon dioxide	28.0		20.0–34.0
Calcium	9.4		8.5–10.6
Phosphorus, Inorganic	3.2		2.5–4.5
Protein, Total	7.0		6.0–8.5
Albumin	4.2		3.2–5.5
Globulin, Total	2.8		1.5–3.8
A/G Ratio	1.5		1.0–2.7
Bilirubin, Total	0.4		0.2–1.2
Bilirubin, Direct	0.2		0.0–0.3
Bilirubin, Indirect	0.2		0.0–0.9
Alkaline Phosphatase	61.0		20.0–140.0
Lactate Dehydrogenase	137.0		0.0–250.0
GGT	16.0		0.0–45.0
AST (SGOT)	22.0		0.0–50.0
ALT (SGPT)	26.0		0.0–55.0
Uric Acid	2.9		2.5–7.5
Iron, Total	115.0		25.0–170.0
Triglycerides	73.0		20.0–160.0
Cholesterol, Total	158.0		<200.0

Complete Blood Count

	Result		Reference Range
White blood cell count	7.5		3.8–10.1
Red blood cell count	4.7		3.9–5.2
Hemoglobin (B)	14.1		12.0–15.6
Hematocrit	41.7		35.0–46.0
MCV	89.6		80.0–100.0
MCH	30.4		27.0–33.0
MCHC	33.9		32.0–36.0
RDW	12.1		9.0–15.0
Platelet count	260.0		130.0–400.0
Neutrophil, SEGS	63.0		40.0–75.0
Lymphocytes	27.7		18.0–47.0
Monocytes	6.5		0.0–12.0
Eosinophils	2.5		0.0–6.0
Basophils	0.3		0.0–2.0

TABLE 15.5
LIFE BALANCES BLOOD TEST EVALUATION: P.W.

	Result	Low	High	Mean	+ or −	Weighted Deviation
BUN/Creat Ratio	18.80	8.00	20.00	14.00	4.80	40.00%
Anion/Cation	10.50	6.00	12.00	9.00	1.50	25.00%
Neutrophils	63.00	40.00	75.00	57.50	5.50	15.71%
Monocytes	6.50	0.00	10.00	5.00	1.50	15.00%
RBC	4.70	3.90	5.20	4.55	.15	11.54%
Hematocrit	41.70	35.00	46.00	40.50	1.20	10.91%
WBC	7.50	3.80	10.10	6.95	.55	8.73%
Hemoglobin	14.10	12.00	15.60	13.80	.30	8.33%
CO_2	28.00	20.00	34.00	27.00	1.00	7.14%
MCH	30.40	27.00	33.00	30.00	.40	6.67%
Globulin	2.80	1.50	3.80	2.65	.15	6.52%
Ca/P Ratio	2.94	2.36	3.40	2.88	.06	5.72%
Iron	115.00	40.00	175.00	107.50	7.50	5.56%
Potassium	4.50	3.50	5.30	4.40	.10	5.56%
Chloride	103.00	95.00	110.00	102.50	.50	3.33%
LDH	137.00	0.00	270.00	135.00	2.00	.74%
Platelet Est.	260.00	130.00	400.00	265.00	− 5.00	− 1.85%
MCV	89.60	80.00	100.00	90.00	− .40	− 2.00%
MCHC	33.90	32.00	36.00	34.00	− .10	− 2.50%
SGPT	26.00	0.00	55.00	27.50	− 1.50	− 2.73%
BUN	15.00	7.00	25.00	16.00	− 1.00	− 5.56%
SGOT	22.00	0.00	50.00	25.00	− 3.00	− 6.00%
Albumin	4.20	3.20	5.50	4.35	− .15	− 6.52%
Calcium	9.40	8.50	10.60	9.55	− .15	− 7.14%
A/G Ratio	1.50	1.00	2.20	1.60	− .10	− 8.33%
Eosinophils	2.50	0.00	6.00	3.00	− .50	− 8.33%
Total Protein	7.00	6.00	8.50	7.25	− .25	− 10.00%
Triglycerides	73.00	20.00	160.00	90.00	− 17.00	− 12.14%
Ionized Calcium	4.16	3.80	4.80	4.30	− .14	− 14.08%
GGT	16.00	0.00	45.00	22.50	− 6.50	− 14.44%
Phosphorus	3.20	2.50	4.50	3.50	− .30	− 15.00%
Alk. Phosphatase	61.00	20.00	140.00	80.00	− 19.00	− 15.83%
Lymphocytes	27.70	18.00	47.00	32.50	− 4.80	− 16.55%
Glucose (Fasting)	85.00	70.00	115.00	92.50	− 7.50	− 16.67%
Chloride/CO_2	3.68	3.24	4.75	3.99	− .31	− 20.74%
Sodium/Potassium	30.44	27.92	38.57	33.25	− 2.80	− 26.33%
Cholesterol	158.00	121.00	304.00	212.50	− 54.50	− 29.78%
Total Bilirubin	.40	.20	1.20	.70	− .30	− 30.00%
Sodium	137.00	135.00	148.00	141.50	− 4.50	− 34.62%
Basophils	.30	0.00	2.00	1.00	− .70	− 35.00%
Creatinine	.80	.70	1.40	1.05	− .25	− 35.71%
Uric Acid	2.90	2.50	7.50	5.00	− 2.10	− 42.00%

Avg. Deviation   14.20%

+ or − Deviation   − 5.80%

TABLE 15.6
LIFE BALANCES BLOOD TEST EVALUATION: P.W.
Continued

Electrolytes	*Deviation*
Sodium	-34.62%
Potassium	5.56%
Chloride	3.33%
CO_2	7.14%
Calcium	-7.14%
Total Deviation	11.56%
+ or –	
Deviation	-5.15%

Renal Function	*Deviation*
BUN	-5.56%
Chloride	3.33%
CO_2	7.14%
Creatinine	-35.71%
Potassium	5.56%
Sodium	-34.62%
Total Deviation	15.32%
+ or –	
Deviation	-9.98%

Liver Function	*Deviation*
SGOT	-6.00%
SGPT	-2.73%
GGT	-14.44%
Total Bilirubin	-30.00%
Alk. Phosphatase	-15.83%
Total Deviation	13.80%
+ or –	
Deviation	-13.80%

Lipids	*Deviation*
Cholesterol	-29.78%
Triglycerides	-12.14%
Total Deviation	20.96%
+ or –	
Deviation	-20.96%

Hematology	*Deviation*
WBC	8.73%
RBC	11.54%
Hemoglobin	8.33%
Hematocrit	10.91%
MCV	-2.00%
MCH	6.67%
MCHC	-2.50%
Platelets	-1.85%
Total Deviation	6.57%
+ or –	
Deviation	4.98%

Diff. WBC	*Deviation*
Neutrophils	15.71%
Lymphocytes	-16.55%
Monocytes	15.00%
Eosinophils	-8.33%
Basophils	-35.00%
Total Deviation	18.12%
+ or –	
Deviation	-5.83%

Ratios	*Deviation*
Anion/Cation	25.00%
Ca/P	5.72%
Na/K	-26.33%
Cl/CO_2	-20.74%
BUN/Creat	40.00%
Total Deviation	23.56%
+ or –	
Deviation	4.73%

Proteins	*Deviation*
Total Protein	-10.00%
Albumin	-6.52%
Globulin	6.52%
A/G Ratio	-8.33%
Total Deviation	7.84%
+ or –	
Deviation	-4.58%

three times a week. She is to salt her food. She will get another blood analysis in sixty days.

The following is a letter she sent after forty-five days of participation in the program:

> For the first time in approximately twenty-two months, I feel like a normal, healthy person again. I am convinced that your system is exactly what has been missing from *my* system. I have been to six different physicians in the past two years trying to find a diagnosis for my constant fatigue and lack of immunity. Initially, antibiotics helped fight some of the symptoms, but with each new episode of illness, the antibiotics did less and less until I finally stopped taking them and started looking in another direction. Your program, within my first three weeks, made dramatic improvements in my health. I'm glad you warned me that I might have days when I felt the same old tiredness, because when those days came, I was mentally prepared and this helped push me on to the next day. Now, forty-nine days into the program, I have *none* of the symptoms I explained in my health questionnaire and I seldom feel tired. After having felt poorly for so long, it's hard to repress myself as I begin to normalize.
>
> Last night I took my first aerobics class in four months and made it through the full hour. I felt great!! My numbers on the day-to-day charts (the smelling test numbers) are consistently growing higher and higher and I have even been able to skip a day . . . a sure sign to me that I'm rapidly improving. The best part of all— my husband and son are so glad to have me back in the family again. I no longer require long naps in the afternoon and I don't have to have ten hours of sleep at night.
>
> I went back and figured out the cost of the two years of medical/prescription treatment, which brought me no relief, and compared those figures to my investment in Life Balances. Actually, there was not much to compare. Life Balances was a fraction of the amount my insurance company was responsible for in that two-

year period. In fact, the cost of Life Balances proved to be the actual cost of the return of my health.

As one of your clients, this is my way of letting you know that you have provided me with a wonderful system that has given me back my health. I'm convinced the longer you are without your health, the more valuable it becomes to you. Remembering all the long days that I was ill, I can't begin to tell you how important your products are to me. Even when I no longer need them on a daily basis, it's comforting to know that I can use my own sensory system to heal myself. Thank you,

P.W.

Disorders of thought, mood, feeling, and perception are chemical tilts, and must be treated with the proper nutrients.

16

The Immune System: Allergies and Sensitivities

Allergies are a useless waste of time. The misery that allergic reactions produce tell you that something irritating is nearby. A rock in your shoe tells you something. The rattle of a rattlesnake tells you danger is close. But why do strawberries taste so good and yet for some, are a deadly poison? Shellfish. Beautiful flowers, a cuddly cat, a friendly dog, or a stuffed toy. The body reacts to a foreign substance and alerts the self to avoid that irritant, whether it is food, contactant, or inhalant. The nature of a distorted body chemistry explains these reactions.

Many have limited the amounts and varieties of their foods because of reactions, discomfort, allergies, or sensitivities—real or imagined. If the body chemistry is properly balanced, however, one can eat, smell, and touch almost anything with impunity. Some people feel that they have fixed allergies, because their allergens have been verified by the RAST, a blood test that seems to be specific for food allergies mediated via gamma globulin E. Usually one can overcome these allergies if the culprit foods are avoided for three to six months, and the body chemistry has been brought into balance. After that abstinence period one would be prudent to consume those foods no more frequently than every four to five days.

Food sensitivities also can be controlled if the body's acidity/alkalinity is controlled. Extra electrolytes act as buffers, and the expected reaction does not occur or it is mild and tolerable.

I used to be sensitive to dairy products manifested as colic, ear infections, bed-wetting, postnasal drip, nose bleeds, migraines, and dandruff. I had all those problems sequentially from infancy on until about three years ago. All of them could be traced to milk consumption. But now because I have balanced my chemistry and I have a better buffering mechanism working, I can drink milk and eat cheese with minimal discomfort—just a little laryngeal phlegm. Maybe these "fixed" reactions to foods are not as permanent as we think. The chemistry of the body can be balanced so that it can handle pollution, allergens, and surly coworkers.

The fact of the allergy, however, is a clue that the victim must change his/her diet and lifestyle. If your body is in perfect balance, allergies—to foods, inhalants, or contactants—will be deprived of practical significance. An allergy, like an infection, basically means that the body is signaling the owner that there is a problem, a slippage. It is quite obvious that the allergic person will avoid the sensitizing food, the rash-producing soap, and the cats causing the sneeze and wheeze. That's a given. If it is a human problem, why doesn't everyone develop these allergies to the same things and to the same degree? If life were fair, we would all get phlegm from milk, like we all bleed when stabbed with a knife.

The Territory

It is the *territory* that determines the type and extent of the allergy. Sure, most people with allergies can point to a relative with a similar response to the environment or some food. Allergists tell me that the majority of the people filing through their offices for periodic testing and desensitizing shots are fair—blue-eyed blondes or green-eyed, freckle-faced, ginger-haired. But African–Americans and Latinos have plenty of allergies, too. No one seems to be immune. Genetics does play a role and certainly is a force to make some susceptible folk fall apart with these allergic reactions when stressors attack.

I just talked to a woman whose three-year-old child is recovering from a six-week bout with whooping cough. Now the child has a watery nose, and a persistent night cough. I asked about sneezing, nose rubbing, and if the discharge was clear. Answers: "Yes, yes, yes." This poor little thing has developed an allergy to some inhalant. They have a cat, there is house dust, and she uses a down comforter. The girl also drinks milk. Treatment: stop all dairy products, get the cat out, clean up her room—make it as bare as a monk's cell. (She will sleep in the bathtub with suitable cotton padding for a few nights to see if the symptoms will disappear. The bathroom is the least dusty room of the house.) The RAST determines if the IGE (Immune Globulin E) is the reactive part of her blood. The animal danders and the house dust will show up on this test, but the food sensitivities will not. (Allergies will; sensitivities do not.) I think we can piece together what has happened. The stress of the disease has exhausted the child's immune system. Her body is saying, "I've had it. Now build me up."

Hans Selye

Hans Selye knew these things back in the 1930s. A stressor, specific or nonspecific, has the capacity of 1) stimulating the adrenal glands to the point of exhaustion; 2) making the thymus and the lymph nodes discharge their white cells; and 3) producing stomach ulcers and hemorrhages. (He called this response the General Adaptive Syndrome: "the nonspecific response of the body to any demand.") If we can eliminate stress, calm down the symptoms that have already told us the child is vulnerable, and build up these tired tissues, she should be her old happy, healthy, vigorous, nonallergic self in a couple of months. She will, probably, always be susceptible to such respiratory insults as weather changes, virus epidemics, tobacco, and exhaust fumes. She may need protective supplements all her life.

This problem is a vicious cycle. If the adrenal and lymph tissues are not restored to full, functioning capacity, the night cough, insomnia, and mucous membrane irritation will continue to act as stressors. The disease that tells us she is ill is a stressor that continues to make her sick because of this continual drain to the immune system. The allergy sufferer cannot get well because he is allergic. Antihistaminics may help control the symptoms, but they will not heal the weakened immune system.

If the mother puts this little girl on a limited diet of carrot juice, fish, zucchini, and white rice, the symptoms may be assuaged, but she has not strengthened the glands, the tissues, and the enzymes that will protect her daughter from the next stress, which may be but a minor irritation to most, but would be a major catastrophe to this now-fragile girl.

Any allergy symptoms conceivably are helpful motivators to encourage one to shore up a truncated immune system. The blood test reveals a possible anemia and a general nutrient deficiency. The total protein, albumin and globulin, are usually below the mean. (Protein is necessary to build antibodies.) Calcium, GGT (a marker for magnesium), serum iron, and potassium are usually in the low range of normal but well below the mean. The eosinophils, a clue about allergies, is usually up at least to 5 percent of the white blood cell count.

The key heroes in controlling allergies and bolstering immunity are vitamins C, A, pantothenic acid, B_6, and B_3. Despite a plugged nose, most allergic people like the smell of these nutrients and might need them two or three times daily.

The amino acid supplements should be used for a month or so that they will be absorbed and help build the glands and the globulins. The efficacy of the intestinal lining cells cannot be trusted to digest and absorb the food proteins needed for anabolism. A few B_{12} shots might be considered here. B_{12} is especially needed for rapidly growing cells, like the lining of the gut.

The incidence of these sensitivities is increasing due to contactants and inhalants but also to food. The chemical pollution of our air, water, and food is a factor, but few authorities have addressed the common villain here, the growing alkalinity of our soil and, consequently, our food. As the earth ages, it becomes more alkaline. Farmers find it cost effective to put potash, phosphates, and nitrates on the soil. The plants grow well, but they are missing some of the micronutrients that make the food worth our eating. When we eat alkaline foods, we tend to become alkaline. The sodium and potassium tends to rise and the anion/cation score would go up.

If people are too alkaline, or too acidic, the minerals are not at the right pH range to make them soluble and available for use by the enzymes.

If you have discovered from your chemical screen that you are alkaline (or acidic), you can remove some of the guesswork from your allergy control. Here is how this works. A lady I know came from the garden last spring sputtering, coughing, sneezing with bloodshot eyes and a watery nose. She was a faucet. I asked

Kitkoski what would be the best thing to do as she does not do well with antihistamines. The chemist recommended six tablets of the ammonium chloride (the acidifier), as he remembered that she was quite alkaline. The pills smelled good to her (like vanilla), and in twenty minutes her allergy symptoms were 90 percent gone. No side effect except a little queasy stomach from the salt load.

Thus demonstrates the magic of following the chemical rules of living.

AIDS

Allopathic control is limited to the use of AZT, and DDI. A vaccine may be out soon. Alternative health doctors use intravenous vitamin C and insist that their patients use no street drugs and they must stop smoking, and eat a nourishing diet. The following have been helpful to boost the immune system: *Echinacea*, aloe vera, essential fatty acids, *Lomatium disectum*, licorice, Saint John's wort, *Chilidonium*, *Astragalus*, *Ligustrum*.

AIDS
A Case Study

The client, LS, was thirty-two years old when he was diagnosed as having the AIDS Related Complex (ARC) in 1983, because of malaise, dizziness, nausea, body aches, extreme fatigue, low-grade fever, diarrhea, persistent swollen lymph nodes, and a history of oral thrush (candidiasis). Cytomegalic blood test was positive. Hepatitis core antibody was positive. He returned to work part time. In 1984 he had a positive HIV test for the AIDS antibody. The doctor gave him little hope that he would ever recover.

In 1984 he had treatment from a Regenesis body worker; the therapy is a form of acupressure. It helped the pain and improved the energy. In January 1985 he started using the healing philosophy of Dr. Louise Hay (*You Can Heal Yourself*. Santa Monica, CA: Hay House, 1987). He has been going to the study group since then. However, in July 1985, he collapsed at work. His doctors said he had to stop work.

(continued on page 206)

(continued from page 205)
He then was treated by a homeopathic doctor in the fall of 1985. He discovered the Life Balances program that winter and went to Spokane in October of 1986. From then until 1988 he followed the Life Balances program faithfully. "Most of my ARC symptoms have disappeared, my lymph nodes have decreased in size, my blood work looks better, and I have more energy."

TABLE 16.1
ABBREVIATED BLOOD TEST EVALUATIONS: L.S.

	July, '85	Oct., '85	Nov., '85	Jan., '86
Sodium	3.85%	− 34.0%	− 34.00%	− 26.00%
Calcium	7.14%	− 7.0%	2.38%	− 2.38%
GGT	− 20.70%	− 13.0%	− 22.00%	− 10.00%
Cholest	134.00%	73.0%	144.00%	184.00%
Triglyc	337.90%	70.0%	209.00%	197.00%
WBC	5.40%	6.9%	11.50%	− 19.00%

	Oct., '86	Nov., '86	Dec., '86	Jan., '87
Sodium	26.00%	− 19%	− 3.05%	− 19.2%
Calcium	0.00%	− 7%	30.95%	− 16.0%
GGT	− 28.00%	− 30%	− 13.00%	− 19.0%
Cholest	96.00%	208%	175.00%	126.0%
Triglyc	222.00%	167%	109.00%	97.0%
WBC	− 26.00%	− 10%	48.00%	77.0%

	Feb., '87	Aug., '87	Oct., '87	Jan., '88
Sodium	− 3.80%	− 19.00%	26.90%	− 19%
Calcium	− 11.90%	− 20.00%	0.00%	− 7%
GGT	− 23.80%	− 6.30%	15.00%	− 14%
Cholest	219.00%	167.00%	128.00%	233%
Triglyc	169.00%	465.00%	484.00%	206%
WBC	13.00%			− 10%

(continued on page 207)

(continued from page 206)

	Feb., '88	*Apr., '88*	*Jun., '88*	*Aug., '88*
Sodium	− 26.90%	− 3.8%	− 26.90%	− 26.90%
Calcium	− 30.90%	11.9%	− 7.10%	− 7.10%
GGT	25.00%	− 28.4%	− 36.10%	− 25.30%
Cholest	88.40%	192.4%	150.00%	91.60%
Triglyc	271.60%	182.0%	162.00%	163.70%
WBC	− 30.00%	− 26.9%	− 14.60%	− 13.00%

	Sept. '88
Sodium	11.50%
Calcium	2.38%
GGT	− 10.00%
Cholest	115.60%
Triglyc	116.2%
WBC	− 20.70%

He wrote this in October 1988, ''My energy level is not back to normal yet as I require a lot of sleep and must stop during the day to take naps, but it is much better than it used to be. I still experience muscle and body aches but this also is not as severe as it used to be. I also get skin rashes mostly on my face. I feel that the Life Balances program has greatly enhanced my life, health, and well-being.''

His blood tests reveal the connection between his symptoms and the changes in his chemistry.

Another AIDS case. "D"

I wish I had understood the connection between skewed chemistry and disease onset forty years ago. I had little more than my medical education to fall back on. That information was worthless in my dealings with my son, D, the milk-sensitive boy who had colic, ear infections, bed-wetting, and pimples. I thought that if milk was that much of a poison to him, it was better to proscribe it and assume if he had nourishing foods, he would get enough calcium. There is calcium in many vegetables, some nuts and a few fruits, isn't there? I also assumed that there was enough calcium in the topsoil from which the plants were growing. He was, however, always a little smaller and a little thinner than his siblings. That should have alerted me that something was amiss.

(continued on page 208)

(continued from page 207)
He broke his right femur skiing at age eleven. The orthopedist, reading the film, said, "Well, there's the break, but see how dense the bone is. Shows he's drinking his milk."

My response, "He's had maybe a quart a year for the last ten years." (I found out since then that ⅓ of bone calcium has to be lost before it will be detected by a standard X ray.)

A homosexual, he became a classics scholar with a degree in Greek studies, wrote books, and articles. When he was about thirty-three years old he had his first bout with pneumonia, his HIV test became positive, and he started the Life Balances program in earnest.

His blood tests showed constant low levels of calcium and sodium despite swallowing all the table salt (2 to 3 teaspoons/day) he could tolerate and 500 to 1000 mg of calcium tablets. Every one of the bottles in the kit had only a slight odor for him (score 4) so he needed everything, even the—to most people—evil-smelling betaine HCl.

His T-cell count (normal is around 1000), an indication of the strength of the immune system, slowly dropped and for the last year of his life it hovered around 10 or less. He insisted on taking AZT, which has now been found to be "safe" if one is not sick, but may hasten the decline of those persons with AIDS. I believe the AZT worked against the Life Balances program. I gave him B_{12} shots (1 ml intramuscularly) every few days; that seemed to slow down the tendency to anemia. He had about ten spots of the Kaposi's sarcoma scattered over his body. Inhalations of pentamidine were mildly helpful in slowing the progress of his pneumocystis pneumonia but could not reverse it. I tried a few injections of intravenous vitamin C, but it only stalled the inevitable decline for a few days or weeks. He lost weight and was skin and bones at the end. His brain was active, bright and alert till the last few days. He had no diarrhea.

I learned how to use hydrotherapy from my naturopathic friends. A treatment takes forty-five minutes and is a mixture of electrical stimulation with alternate hot and cold towels on his chest and abdomen, front and back. After a treatment he would not cough for twelve hours.

It is known that sodium and potassium—under the direction of calcium and magnesium—control the cell wall "traffic." The virus seems to have an easy time spreading from one cell to another if the serum levels of sodium and calcium are not optimal. (Recall that medieval food handlers salted meat to prevent spoilage. Salty chicken soup will slow the invasion of germs into human meat. Epidemics of infectious disease are more likely to hit those with low serum sodium.)

We could not save him but we were able to prolong his life and make him comfortable for his last twelve to eighteen months despite a nonexistent T-cell count.

Allergies

The allopathic allergist will help the patient control contacts, foods, and the environment. Skin tests are the basis of the investigation. Desensitizing shots help control the symptoms. Antihistaminics are used for temporary control. Naturopathic doctors find that the Vega test is valuable to discover food sensitivities. Homeopathy can help. Vitamins C, B_6, B_{12}, pantothenic acid, bioflavonoids, and E can help. Herbalists use nettles, adrenalinum, *Magnesia phosphorica*, lymph, *Apis mellifica*, hydrastis, gentian, garlic, fenugreek.

Asthma

Allergist will do the above investigation for allergies, and use cortisone, cromolyn, inhalants, and epinephrine shots for temporary control. Natural methods include B_{12} shots, B_6, C, magnesium, no milk, no wheat diet with emphasis on vegetarianism. Relaxation, homeopathy can help. Herbalists use adrenalinum, *Carbo vegetabilis*, lung, *Arsenicum album*, *Bryonia alba*, camphora, *Atropa belladonna*, *Natrum muriaticum*, *Natrum suphuricum*, alfalfa, ephedra, garlic, lobelia, fenugreek, wild cherry, pleurisy root, mullein, horehound, and capsicum.

Bacterial Infections

The standard allopathic control is to use antibiotics. If repeated infections, the immune system is evaluated. Natural control can be achieved with vitamin C (1000 mg every hour), *Echinacea*, thymus gland, *Hypericum*, berberis, goldenseal, myrrh, oregano, garlic, onions, tree tea oil, vitamin A and zinc, dandelion root, chaparral, burdock root, licorice root, and sarsaparilla.

Cancer

Allopathic control is limited to surgery, chemotherapy, and X-radiation. Natural methods try to boost the immune system once the tumor has been excised. Twenty grams of vitamin C per day is standard, along with A, Hoxey formula, Essiac formula (burdock, sheep sorrel, turkey rhubarb, slippery elm).

Candidiasis (Yeast Infection)

Allopathic control consists of the use of antiyeast drugs: Nystatin, Nizoral. Natural methods include no sugar, and curtail the use of antibiotics and birth-control pills. Vitamins C, A, *Echinacea*, usnea, green walnut, *Lactobacillus acidophilus*.

Ear Infections

Allopathic methods are based on the use of antibiotics, and some allergy control. Most alternative doctors will stop the use of dairy products, and add vitamins A, E, C, zinc, yellow dock, goldenseal, hypericum oil, mullein eardrops, *Echinacea*, and bioflavonoids.

Eczema

Allopathic doctors use cortisone ointments, food elimination, and antihistaminics. A more natural approach by alternative doctors employs vitamin A, zinc, the B vitamins, selenium, omega-6 oil, flax oil, sulfur, garlic, and lecithin along with the herbs: Aloe vera, burdock, kelp, slippery elm, red clover, silybum, berberis, dandelion, chickweed. They will stop dairy products, and proscribe wheat, eggs, sugar, and chocolate. A liver cleanse is worthwhile. Homeopathy will help. Pantothenic acid and calendula creams are soothing.

Lupus Erythematosis

The allopathic approach is to use cortisone and other antiinflammatory drugs. A more natural approach would be to build the immune system with A, beta-carotene, pantothenic acid, B_{12}, E, C, zinc, calcium, magnesium, Thymus gland, cysteine, methionine, omega-3 fatty acids. Looking for food sensitivities may be rewarding. Many have low stomach acid.

Urinary Tract Infections

Allopathic treatment is usually just antibiotics, but that frequently leads to yeast infections. A more natural method is one or all of the following: vitamins C, A, B_6, Betaine HCl, and cranberry juice. Acidifying the urine is important as germs do not live in acid urine. These herbs will help: watermelon seed tea, *Uva ursi*, goldenrod tea, juniper berries, nettle, marshmallow root, alfalfa, parsley, corn silk, pipsissewa.

Virus Infections

Most infections are due to viruses. "It's the virus that is going around." A few antivirals are helpful if a patient is very sick: Virex, Acyclovir. Safe treatment by alternative doctors includes vitamin C, 1000 mg every hour; echinacea, thymus extract, *Lomatium disectum*, osha root, hypericum, ligustium, and astragalus.

17

Amino and Fatty Acid Supplements

Supplemental Amino Acids

Vitamins and minerals cannot do their various jobs unless the amino acids are available to make the enzymes, the catalysts of all body functions. About twenty times the quantity of the amino acids are needed for each unit of the vitamins and minerals just to maintain these enzymes. The plasma concentrations of each type of amino acid is maintained at a constant value, except after several weeks of severe starvation, when stored fats have been burned up, then the amino acids of the blood are called upon to become oxidized for energy.

If the blood tests show low protein (albumin and globulin are both below the mean) either from eating protein-deficient foods or from malabsorption, the following deficiency signs may be present: edema, nausea, dizziness, poor coordination, overall weakness, anemia, cataracts, lowered resistance to infection, cuticles tear easily, low hormone levels, impaired growth, muscle wasting. The diet should be adequate to supply the protein needs of the body. Many people have limited their intake because of food sensitization reactions, but they may be jeopardizing their health as protein is needed for immunity, allergy control, and all the rest of the metabolism. Using amino acids on a temporary basis for convalescence or for those with extremely weak digestive abilities is prudent.

Amino acids are the basic protein building blocks. They are needed to make the brain's neurotransmitters, the liver and intestinal enzymes, and all the other enzyme systems of the different cells. Because they are so basic, they are not considered foreign substances by the body and, hence will not trigger an allergic reaction. Human intestinal digestion of plant and animal protein is supposed to break down the protein molecules to these basic, nonallergic amino acid units for absorption into the system where the liver puts them together as human protein. That process may not be complete, so therefore, reactions may occur to these incompletely broken down proteins. The body's immune system may think it is a foreign invader.

Some eight amino acids must be supplied by the diet. They are called essential. The other 14—there may be more—can be manufactured by the body from these eight. If these eight are not supplied in the proper amounts, or there is some pathway block in the protein synthesis, essential enzymes cannot be manufactured. For example, L-tyrosine is an amino acid and needs iodine to become thyroxin, the thyroid hormone. Without iodine there is no hormone; without tyrosine, there is no hormone. They are interdependent.

That is why eating good food and taking extra vitamins and minerals may not be enough to "prime the pump" of the body's metabolic fires; amino acid therapy is ideal for the person who has tried everything and is still sick and tired. It can control obesity in many. This is the reason that many nutrition-oriented doctors use amino acid supplements for a month or two to get these enzymes working.

Capsules of amino acids are readily absorbed and will quickly team up with the appropriate vitamins and minerals to be used to duplicate the genetic code (as in cell division), to form muscles, connective tissue, metabolize hormones, form enzymes, and produce neurotransmitters. Once the machinery is operating smoothly, these amino acid supplements can be discontinued and sensible eating habits will maintain the physiology. Continued use is fine, but can be expensive. They are utilized best if taken on an empty stomach.

Threonine is important in fat metabolism, and is low in those on a vegetarian diet. People who have little are often irritable, hard to get along with. Suggested: 350 to 3,000 mg daily.

L-Glutamic Acid detoxifies ammonia, which is common in candida sufferers. It aids brain metabolism, often controls symptoms of hypoglycemia, and, thus, is a standby in the treatment of alcoholism. L-Glutamine passes through the blood-brain barrier and becomes L-Glutamic acid in the brain and is used as a fuel. Suggested: 500 to 2,000 mg daily.

L-Carnitine will reduce some of the risk for elevated fats and cholesterol in the blood. It can improve heart muscle exercise tolerance as it facilitates the transport of fatty acids into the energy center of the muscle cells. It can dilate the coronary blood vessels and even lower blood pressure. L-Lysine and L-Methionine will produce L-Carnitine, but an enzyme malfunction may not allow enough to be manufactured. Suggested: 350 to 1,000 mg daily between meals.

L-Phenylalanine is a precursor to L-Tyrosine, which in turn makes L-Dopa and ultimately becomes dopamine and norepinephrine and epinephrine. Are all considered stimulants; they elevate mood and make one more alert and ambitious. Depression-prone people might find this cheaper and safer than taking mood-elevating drugs. It also curbs appetite as it releases cholecystokinin, which subdues the foraging center of the brain. Suggested: 300 to 2,000 mg daily between meals.

Taurine is most important for those prone to heart problems. It has regulatory effect on membrane excitability of heart muscle and nerve cells, and on the central nervous system as well. Suggested: 200 to 1,000 mg daily between meals.

Tryptophan is the precursor to serotonin, which minimizes the brain's reaction to the stressors in the environment. It calms anxiety, lifts depression, and counteracts insomnia. It also reduces vulnerability to heart diseases. It can act as an appetite control; it decreases the desire for carbohydrates. Vitamin C, B_6, and B_3 are necessary to convert tryptophan to serotonin.

("It is possible that some overweight or depressed people overconsume dietary carbohydrates, using these foods as though they were antidepressant drugs to increase their serotonin levels." Richard Wurtman, M.D., 1987.) Suggested: 500 to 1,500 mg daily.

Along with these special ones for the specific problems, doctors usually have their patients take amino acid blends containing the twenty-one or twenty-two amino acids daily to prevent an imbalance. Suggested: 300 to 700 mg daily between meals.

How do you know if you need supplemental amino acids? Notice on the laboratory printout if your albumin is below the mean. Albumin is an indicator of sufficient protein in the diet. The globulin is manufactured chiefly by the liver, but the liver needs protein (amino acids) to produce globulin, a key substance in immunity. Some people are eating sufficient protein, but their digestive enzymes—chiefly stomach acid—are not sufficient to break the protein down into the basic, absorbable amino acids.

Supplemental Fatty Acids

Some fat is important in the diet as a source of energy. Furthermore, it satisfies hunger better than other foods. People who adhere to the Pritikin diet, which contains only 10 percent fat, complain of being extremely hungry. Fats also are important for the proper absorption of minerals, and fatty acids and their products are crucial ingredients of all membranes, like the cell walls. If you don't get enough essential fatty acids, the mucous membrane of the intestinal tract becomes more permeable and undigested foods and toxins may enter the bloodstream (the leaky gut). Lipids account for 70 percent of the materials used to construct the brain. The word "essential" is used because people must have them to survive. Essential fatty acids are used to build structural lipids in a similar way as essential amino acids build protein. Particular molecules, such as octacosanal may actually build the myelin sheath around nerve cells.

Fatty acid molecules are carbon chains or various lengths with a nonpolar methyl end (CH_3) and a carboxyl (COOH) end, which is a weak acid. The fatty acids may be saturated because all the carbon atoms have all the outer rings filled with hydrogen atoms. These saturated fats are oxidized by the body to provide energy, calories, and heat, but they also serve as insulation under the skin and around organs, and as part of the structure of cell membranes. The unsaturated fatty acids have double bonds between some of the carbon atoms as hydrogen atoms have not occupied all the outer rings. These make prostaglandins, create electrical potential, and provide structure and fluidity of the cell membranes.

These prostaglandins have hormonelike regulating functions: regulate the stickiness of the blood platelets, play a role in clotting diseases (heart attacks, stroke, embolism, phlebitis, and arterial disease), help control blood pressure, regulate inflammatory conditions, exert some control over sodium and water retention via the kidneys, are involved with the immune system. They affect every cell and organ in the body.

The American Heart Association suggests that we reduce fat consumption from 40 percent of total calories (a typical diet) to less than 30 percent. Dietary fats should include polyunsaturated fatty acids (vegetable and seed oils such as safflower, sunflower, corn), some monounsaturated (olive oil) as well as a minimal amount from saturated fats (in meat, milk products, eggs, and some warm-water foods such as shrimp and crab). What should be avoided are the partially hydrogenated fats that are found in many bakery goods as well as in margarine and shortenings.

"Good" or "essential" fatty acids (EFA) cannot be manufactured by the body. These EFAs are cis-linoleic and alpha linolenic acids, which are the precursors to yet other substances call prostaglandins E1 and E3, respectively, or PGE1 and PGE3 for short. These particular PGEs tend to lower the tryglycerides (fat) and LDL cholesterol (dangerous kind) and raise the HDL cholesterol (safer kind) in the blood. Further, a lack of these PGEs may cause any or all of the following symptoms: brittle nails, dry skin, dandruff, eczema, acne, extreme thirst, hyperactivity, premenstrual syndrome, asthma, arthritis, high blood pressure, coronary heart disease, and obesity.

A source of one of the EFAs—cis-linoleic acid, or cis-LA—is cold-pressed vegetable or seed oil (corn, safflower, sunflower, cottonseed). Your body supplies an enzyme that makes gamma linolenic acid (GLA) from cis-LA and this in turn becomes PGE1. (Human breast milk supplies GLA directly, but if you are an adult, this source dried up long ago.) If, as a child, you were hyperactive, fair, had eczema, asthma, and were unusually thirsty, you may have a genetic deficiency of the enzyme that helps make GLA. You can stimulate the production of that enzyme by taking supplements of C, E, A, B_3, B_6, biotin, beta-carotene, zinc, and magnesium. Most participants in the program with these symptoms find these supplements smell good to them. If these are not helpful, then you might try evening primrose oil, a good source of GLA. The body then can make PGE1 easily.

A source of the other EFA—alpha linolenic acid, or ALA—is flaxseed oil as well as some nuts and legumes. ALA also requires that enzyme mentioned above to turn it into eicosapentaenoic acid (EPA), which in turn becomes PGE3. This EPA can be obtained at the health food store, but eating some cold-water fish such as salmon, herring, cod, or mackerel twice a week might be sufficient. The body turns it into PGE3.

The saturated fats from meat, milk, eggs, and freshwater fish contain arachidonic acid (AA). This stimulates the production of PGE2, which leads to inflammation, increased platelet aggregation, and water retention. It is more likely to increase the production of LDL cholesterol, considered to be the more dangerous form of cholesterol. Some saturated fats are required in the diet, but not in the quantities that are normally eaten in the U.S. These saturated fatty acids are straight chains, without bends and are slow to react with other substances. Saturated fats have a higher melting point: they become harder at room temperature and are more likely to become sticky in the bloodstream.

Unsaturated fats have kinks in their molecules that prevent them from stacking together and aggregating as saturated fats do. They melt at much lower temperatures and are liquid in the body. (Cold-water fish have these fats; that is why they are not stiff at deep ocean temperature.)

The *cis* configuration has two hydrogen atoms missing on each side of the double bond. This forms a gap. The fatty acid molecule kinks at that area to fill in the gap. This provides the integrity of these structural lipids. It also serves to lock in sulphur molecules that comprise half of all cellular membranes, and some of the internal structures of the cell. This bending of the long molecules is important for the cell wall structure. *Trans* fats, on the other hand, are created by the hydrogenation of natural fatty acids. Margarine is an example. This manufacturing process straightens out the fats by inserting hydrogen into the carbons where the double bonds allowed the chain to bend. The trans-fatty acid then becomes straight, becomes hard at room temperature, and can stack up in your vessels. They should be avoided for cooking and eating. We must, therefore, avoid margarine, hydrogenated fat, processed foods, and heated or fried fats or foods containing them.

Clumping of blood cells has its root cause in the propensity for saturated fats to lie close together in a rigid structure and to be solid like candles. To reverse the stiffness produced by the straight chains of long-chain saturated fatty acids, one should consume long-chain polyunsaturated fatty acids with their twists to counteract those stacked rigid saturated-with-hydrogen chains. Unsaturated fats, with their lower melting point, do not stack up like pages of a book, as they are liquid at body temperature, and give the cell wall fluidity. This is at the very basis of getting nutrients into the cells. Cells must be able to trap and hold the molecules that are the doorways to permit nutrients to enter and waste products to exit.

To help heal the nervous system in those hurt by cerebral palsy, muscular dystrophy, multiple sclerosis, myasthenia gravis, and brain injury, the essential fatty acids, amino acids, vitamins, and minerals must be able to get through the barrier between the brain capillaries and the brain itself. This blood-brain barrier is a selective filter and is mostly electrical at the surface—accepting unipolar or dipolar molecules. The metal ions involved in the process of passage through the barrier will effect an acid/base change. This change will then cause a change in the radius of the atoms of the elements so that they will move through the barrier. Thus all nutrients must be in the right balance at the right time. (Much of this information comes from Dr. Patricia Kane.)

Dr. Charles Bates, Ph.D., wrote the book *Essential Fatty Acids and Immunity in Mental Health* in 1987. He studied blood samples of Native Americans on Vancouver Island, B.C. and in eastern Washington. For centuries the Indians in the eastern part of the state enjoyed salmon as a staple in their diets, but when the Columbia River dams wiped out most of the salmon, they developed schizophrenia at double the North American average (plus arthritis, diabetes, alcoholism, migraine, obesity, and depression). Eskimos, Welsh, Scots, and Scandinavians are similarly affected with these diseases. They apparently are lacking the enzyme that helps produce an essential fatty acid. If it is not in their diet, they will get sick.

Rule: Rotate your diet. Do not eat the same things each day. Eliminate fried foods. Avoid all margarines, refined salad, and cooking oils, and partially hydrogenated vegetable and seed oils.

Instead, use cold-pressed vegetable and seed oils, olive oil, and flaxseed oil. Dairy products can be tolerated if mixed with the program's electrolyte solution. Consume a variety of low fat meat, fowl, fish, vegetables, whole grains, salads with some vinegar.

HAVE A GOOD LIFE!

Summary

Your body is wonderfully made. However, it requires constant, intelligent care: optimal fuel, safe fluids, positive social interaction, adequate rest, and appropriate exercise. Our ancestors did all these supportive things automatically, naturally, and easily because there were few choices. Those ancients had no strong, toxic drugs when they were sick. They had wine, witchcraft, and supportive relatives. Your grandparents worked hard physically so they did not need exercise machines. Families ate, played, and prayed together and so had a sense of security and belonging. There was ample fish for the fishermen, abundant trees for the loggers, and enough land for the farmers. Most had a garden with fresh, pesticide-free food. The water was pure until it became contaminated with lead or rat feces.

Now we have store-bought food and store-bought teeth. We eat impoverished foods that give us impoverished bodies. Diseases of degeneration are taking us in our thirties and forties instead of in our eighties and nineties. Alzheimer's disease was a rare problem in 1900, but is hitting many of us after ages fifty or sixty years.

How do we get well, stay well, live a long, pain-free life with no major diseases? Is it possible to live until one hundred and still be able to feed and clothe oneself? Yes, but you must educate yourself about health and diet. Your mother may not have known how that was done because *her* mother only knew about boiling vegetables until they were gray and took the meat off the stove when she smelled smoke.

Although most doctors are motivated enough to read the medical literature, much of that information is the distillation of the research paid for by drug companies. Huge sums of money are required to bring a new drug to the marketplace. And to protect their investment they must sell, sell, sell—which is good business but not necessarily good medicine.

But doctors, whether they are allopathic, naturopathic, chiropractic, osteopathic, or whatever are supposed to be teachers.

Perhaps the patients, the clients, the sick, and helpless can force the doctors to fulfill their traditional role as educator. If a woman is told that she needs estrogen or progesterone because she is a woman and is forty-five years old, that woman should ask, "What is the evidence? Where are the tests that show I am deficient?" Lab work is getting more sophisticated and accurate. If the doctor suggests a skin patch for the transdermal absorption of the hormone, has he evaluated the woman's circulation and blood pressure? If the skin is cold, the hormones may not get through. If the woman gets a shot of the hormone, maybe it will be too much. A complete blood test must be done to evaluate the electrolyte balance and the body's ability to absorb dermatologically, intramuscularly, or orally.

If the doctor is adamant about treating your cholesterol level, which is hovering at 240 mg percent, you might ask on what information he/she is basing his/her concern. Surely he has seen in the medical literature that although the cholesterol levels of Americans have come down 6 percent in the last ten years, the triglyceride levels have moved up about 6 to 12 percent. The alkaline/acid ratio has been altered over this same period of time; alkalinity is on the rise. That one fact is the reason behind the general increase in the incidence of hypertension in the U.S. Cholesterol has some hydrogen in its molecule that contributes to acidity (acidity helps to reduce blood pressure), while tryglycerides have hydroxyl (OH) endings that encourage alkalinity and elevated blood pressure and encourage atherosclerosis. The medical profession is trading off the vague risk of one disease (Reduce the Cholesterol!) with the known incidence of two or three other problems.

The number of kids who are hyperactive and academically dysfunctional is increasing, and not from a Ritalin deficiency. They are getting too many nitrates from preservatives that extend the shelf life of some foods. Does your child's doctor know this? He would if he obtained a complete blood test and scanned it carefully for evidence of nutrient deficiencies and alkalinity. Did you ask your doctor how he knows a stimulant drug is going to help your squirrely kid? This child is probably not getting the proper nutrients to his brain, and is probably low in calcium and magnesium despite drinking much milk. He cannot sit still because his brain cannot make enough of the neurotransmitters that will allow him to focus on the task at hand and follow directions. The evidence is there and waiting for intelligent people to see the obvious.

Why is crime on the increase? Why do people need to take street drugs? These are sick people mentally and physically, but basically nutritionally. The next time you drive through that part of your town inhabited by those who cannot function well in our society, look at their wasted bodies, their sallow complexions. Most real alcoholics have wasted buttocks because their nutrient-poor diets force their bodies to take what nutrients are lying around. They need nutrients together with psychological support from social agencies.

Many runners run because they only feel well while running. They certainly get a lift from the temporary surge of endorphins, but many run because their circulation is so poor that they have to move fast to get some blood and oxygen to their bodies and especially their brains. They must be encouraged to eat a more nourishing diet and increase their salt and fluid intake to move their blood pressure up to a more normal 120 over 80. Life Balances shows them how.

Consumer advocates have helped to slow down the rape of the environment. Advocacy groups have made the government and business accountable for improving our health. Ranchers now give us leaner, better beef. Consumers have made the government regulate lead and pollution in exhausts and water. Grocery managers offer us healthier foods. We must now make our health-care providers accountable for our health by educating us to the chemical ways of the body. You give the history and the urine sample. The blood is drawn. Does the doctor really look at it for the evidence of a chemical tilt that explains your symptoms? Or are you just content to accept the prescription for a diuretic, an antibiotic, a tranquilizer, or an antihistaminic because you don't want to hurt your doctor's feelings?

Go back to the lifestyle of a couple of generations ago. People sat down for meals, laughed, and ate nutrient-rich foods because they could trust the farmers' methods of raising the crops. We had milk, eggs, real butter, meat, vegetables, fruit in season, and whole-grain foods that still had the vitamins and minerals. The blood tests show that most of us are not getting salt, milk, and vinegar in a balanced ratio. True, the milk should be modified by suitable dilution with the electrolyte solution to make the valuable nutrients in the milk available for human consumption and absorption.

We must persuade doctors to work with patients to find the chemical anomalies that explain deviations from health. They cannot just treat our symptoms. That method is no longer acceptable. Causes must be explained *and* understood.

An Invitation to Health Care Providers

The Life Balances Health Program (LB) is specifically designed to allow you to be more helpful to your patients. LB will complement your practice as it is based on the immutable laws of chemistry. The company's founder, John Kitkoski, used existing and ongoing medical studies, reference material from a wide variety of scientific sources, and the Med-Com Network (a computer database that contains medical and scientific research from around the world). He then fit together the methodology that is now the Life Balances Health Program. This process took more than twenty years to assemble, prove, and fine tune.

Life Balances is compatible with your practice methods. It is *not* a substitute for your own proven methods of practice and your long-held beliefs. It will, however, give you added confidence when you advise your patients what they should eat, and what supplements they need to take. It puts accountability where it belongs. If a patient is well, the program will maintain health. If the patient is sick, he/she will get well faster, and often with a minimum of drugs. Doctor means teacher: you will be able to educate your patients toward a healthy lifestyle.

Medical doctors are skilled at prescribing drugs and performing surgery. Chiropractors know that adjustments will relieve pain and alleviate diseases. Naturopathic doctors have several treatment modalities to treat their patients safely. Helpful though these methods are, those patients so treated will return to sickness if no attention is paid to the basic rules of chemistry. The LB program is designed to locate and replace the missing elements in the body *before* a diagnosable disease occurs.

If a disease is already established, the program works in conjunction with existing treatment by replacing the deficient nutrients. You cannot get that patient well unless the acid/base balance is corrected, ratios are optimal, and nutrient densities and deficiencies are returned to near normal. If your patient's chemistry is not in proper balance, his personality, energy, memory, and general health will suffer.

We have proof that a good, balanced diet does not supply all of a person's needs. Stress affects body chemistry. Pollution requires the body to use extra nutrients to detoxify the poisons in our food, water, and air. The need for minerals and vitamins varies depending on the events of the day and the foods eaten. LB research shows that the balanced body chemistry necessary to fight disease or restore health is not produced by so-called one-a-day or multivitamins. They may even increase levels of elements that the body may have in excess already. Balance cannot be obtained when one adds 100 percent of the ingredients. The more one adds of all the ingredients, the more unbalanced the body becomes. The excessively ingested ones rise to toxic levels, and just because they may be water soluble does not mean they will wash out in the urine or stool. Only by increasing the intake of deficient elements, and restricting the use of excessive vitamins and minerals will the balance be achieved. The LB program removes the guesswork from nutritional supplementation.

The diet for a steelworker is different from the diet for a quiet shut-in. The diet for an ectomorph (like Olive Oyl) with a short intestinal tract is different from the diet for an endomorph (like Oliver Hardy) with a long intestinal tract. We are what we absorb and what finally gets into the cells, not necessarily what we swallow. If one is to eat a truly well-balanced diet, a person would have to be accountable for every element that he or she swallows. A well-balanced diet must fit the nutritional needs of that person at that moment in time. If the diet is based on the RDA's nonexistent "normal person," it cannot be well-balanced. If a person eats a dish of oysters, for example, he gets a generous supply of zinc. If he is offered his choice of an apple or an apricot for dessert, he is more likely to choose the apricot. **Reason:** The apple has more zinc than manganese, while the apricot has more manganese than zinc. To balance the body chemistry, our diner reaches for the apricot. Different proportions produce a different end product. Cookies are made from a different recipe than a cake or a pie.

Special diets (grapefruit diets, high-protein diets, strict vegan-vegetarian diets, elimination diets) that restrict certain types of foods create more problems than they solve. If people remove specific foods from their diets, they become deficient in the nutrients present in those foods. On a short-term basis it may ease some symptoms of food sensitivities, but the limited diet will create long-term deficiencies. Everyone needs foods from all food groups regularly to maintain a healthy balance. We all need a variety of foods everyday. The LB program teaches people to rely on their own cravings. "If it sounds, looks, and smells good, you need it." The vitamins and minerals used as part of the program will balance the individual's diet on a daily basis. Supplements are meant to supply the nutrients our wimpy foods do not provide. LB teaches participants to change or vary their diet to rely less on the vitamins and minerals and supply the nutrients by the use of appropriate, wholesome foods, whenever possible.

Treating the symptoms is the present allopathic paradigm for disease control, erroneously called health maintenance. If a person has low tissue magnesium, he might become hyperactive, have heart-rhythm irregularities, or become tense and anxious. Modern treatment demands Ritalin for the former, digitalis for the heart victim, and Valium for the nervous one. Wouldn't it be more logical to replace the missing magnesium? Using the chemical law of definite proportions so important to body chemistry, one has to consider all the elements that work with magnesium. Their values must be measured and appropriate supplements added to the diet.

It is interesting to observe those with low calcium will scarf down milk; the anxious magnesium needers love chocolate; and the warty, vitamin A-deficient people will forage for carrots, sweet potatoes, and parsley.

How to Help Your Patient

All of us were trained as diagnosticians, but, unfortunately, we must wait until a constellation of symptoms coalesces enough to give us that "AHA. You've got . . . !" Then we can write the prescription and put the name of the disease in the patient's chart. Quiet, subtle little changes in the patient's metabolism start without fanfare: vague symptoms of uneasiness, mild aches and pains, odd rashes that come and go, fatigue, not feeling rested after a night's sleep, sense of humor slipping, slight feeling of anxiety for no reason, job, school, home have no appeal, more colds or flu than usual, hair unmanageable—may all appear singly or together.

Based on those symptoms, doctors have no way of establishing a diagnosis except for the wastebaskets of neurasthenia, stress, or hypochondriasis. The physical exam and the blood tests fall within the normal range. But diseases have to start somewhere. We at Life Balances believe we can detect a process on its way to becoming pathology—a disease about to happen. Health practitioners are now in a position to take necessary action to prevent this downhill slide to sickness. Indeed, we have enough science working for us to be able to show that these subtle symptoms can be explained by the deviations from the mean in the blood test. Depletion of nutrient stores cause cellular, metabolic changes. The enzymes that do the work of the body must have the appropriate vitamins and minerals in the proper concentrations. These patients need help, not a pejorative label. They already feel rotten; they do not need our, "There, there, get some rest." (Or, "Why don't you have an affair to lighten things up?")

After you do the examination, and get the history from the patient, the blood is drawn (twenty-four chemical screen plus the CBC) and the test results are fed into the computer for the analysis. Each test is evaluated as to its degree of deviation from the mean of the range of the laboratory's values. The results are evaluated along with the responses to the LB questionnaire and the recommendations are sent to you, the health-care provider. It is impressive how the recommendations fit the symptoms or the disease.

"What is your favorite food?"

"Dairy." Check the calcium level in the blood test; it is usually below the mean.

"Do you like vinegar and pickles?"

"Yes! Do you have some?" Check the blood pressure. It may be up if the sodium level in the blood is above the mean.

Older people tend to produce less hydrochloric acid for stomach digestion of protein. They have dyspepsia, gas, soft nails, and also tend to have elevated blood pressure. Using betaine hydrochloride as a replacement is the treatment, but these people will do better if their chemistry is modified. These achlorhydric folks do not have enough serum iron that acts as a catalyst for the enzyme that splits water into $H+$ and $OH-$. (Young people usually find the smell of betaine disgusting; those without much stomach acid don't mind the smell at all.)

The lower the levels of the nutrients in the body, the sweeter the smell. The worse the smell, the more likely is the nutrient in his/her system. When the computer sorts out the values according to their deviation from the mean, you will see at a glance if the client is nutrient-dense or -deficient.

The body reveals its secrets if we ask the right questions and perform the proper tests. The twenty-four-chemical screen including the CO_2, the serum iron, and the complete blood count is about as accurate as we can get for the price.

We have advanced beyond the nutritional guesswork of a few decades ago. Today we can advise clients what to eat, what supplements to take, and how much—and be accurate.

A Final Note for Those Starting the Program

If you would like to get your blood chemistry done, now that you have completed this much of the book, to see how much common sense the program makes, simply write or call: Life Balances International, 1099 S.W. Columbia Ave., Suite 300, Portland, OR 97201, telephone: (503) 221-1779. The profile and your health history will be thoroughly evaluated. Recommendations for specific supplements to balance the deviation will be made as some values are too far above or below the mean. When the body gets the proper amounts of nutrients in the right ratios for the enzymes to function, health is achieved without drugs.

Participation in the whole program is the best guarantee of success. That includes, along with the blood test and the questionaire, the purchase of the Life Balances Home Health Kit, which includes twenty bottles of individual vitamins and minerals, six dropper bottles, and four bottles of electrolyte concentrate.

We need to make people more accountable for their own health. We must encourage doctors to be more accountable for the patients in their care.

If your scores on the vitamin smells are high (5 to 10), and you eat a lot, you will tend to get diarrhea. If your scores are in the low range (1 to 4), and you don't eat very much, you will tend to be constipated. If you are constipated, eat a meal, then go through the kit. When you are constipated, your body is trying to hold on to the food as long as possible to extract as much of the nutrients as possible from it; it is because you are so deficient.

Many people just starting on the program will feel uncomfortable, or even have pain because the waste materials are being freed and are circulating through the system. It is similar to the sensation when an arm or leg goes to sleep and the blood returning causes pain. This waste material is garbage being pumped out of the tissues. Your circulation has not been good enough in the past to clean out the wastes. You should notice that your hands and feet are warmer.

If you have been sick, you were suffering from an imbalance. The wrong material worked its way into your cells. The nervous system then sends the wrong signals to your body. Muscles then go into spasms, or at least become tense. This damages the tissues. Nutrients cannot get into the cells to repair the damage and eliminate the wastes. Old age is caused by atrophy, which makes the muscles weak and wasted. If the muscles can be relaxed so the proper nutrition can get in and the damaged tissues can be flushed out, the muscles will become strong again. The electrolyte solution relaxes the muscles and puts a balanced solution in place allowing the vitamins and minerals to do their job with the enzymes. Flushing your system with water only helps get some of the garbage out, but until you put in the proper nutrients all you have is a cleaner system.

If you let wet laundry sit in the hamper, it will get moldy. The mold will go all through the clothes as long as the proper conditions are there. Your body is similar; if your sodium level is low, bacteria go all through your body creating congestion and infection. If the laundry had been washed in a sodium solution, the mold would not have grown. To preserve meat, you add salt, for this keeps the bacteria from growing. Our bodies react similarly: we need a balanced chemistry and that includes sodium. Not too much; not too little. Just the right amount.

This seems hard to believe, but it happens. The left side of your body reflects the sodium balance in your system, and the right side the potassium balance. If you are under a lot of stress, your right side will show the change—a limp will be more pronounced, you may drag your foot more, or your right eyelid might droop more than the left—as stress affects the potassium level of the body. The same things happen if your sodium is out of balance, but the changes will be on the left side of your body. Strange but true.

Most people who conscientiously work with the program notice that their arms and legs get softer and larger. This means that the muscles are relaxing. Soon the whole body softens and relaxes. It is a good sign. It is the body saying how good it feels to have some of the tension off so the muscles can relax. If this is happening to you on the program, you will be able to work more efficiently and longer.

Disregard the law of gravity, you will get hurt. Body chemistry is basic to health. Disregard those chemical laws and you will get sick.

AND NOW A WORD FROM CHIEF SEATTLE (1854)

"This we know. The earth does not belong to man; man belongs to the earth. This we know. All things are connected like the blood which unites one family. All things are connected. Whatever befalls the earth befalls the sons of the earth. Man did not weave the web of life; he is merely a strand in it. Whatever he does to the web, he does to himself."

Appendix

Kitkoski has found that he can be of greater help to the client if, along with the blood test analysis, he has the present and past history of the person. For example, he has noticed that people living in the northern areas of the United States are more likely to be alkaline. Different geographical areas have their own disease incidence because of weather, top soil, and pollution problems.

Comprehensive Medical History

Date_____

Name_____ Birth Date____/____/____ Age__

Place of Birth_____

Height_____'_____" Weight_____lbs.

Last blood pressure_____/_____

Occupation_____ Previous Occupation(s)_____
_____
_____

States (Countries) Where You Have Lived_____
_____
_____

Education (Years) High School____ College____ Post-Grad
____

Single____ Married____ Divorced____ Widow(er)____

Hobbies_____

Last Complete Physical Examination (Where & Date)_____
_____

Results_____

CURRENT PROBLEMS

Chief Complaint_____

Describe in Detail_____

_____

Onset_____ How did it begin_____

_____

Under what circumstances does it occur_____

_____

Frequency_____

Severity and Duration/Change_____

_____

What treatment have you had for this problem?_____

_____

Practitioner's name_____

List any additional medical problems with date of onset:

1._____   8._____
2._____   9._____
3._____   10._____
4._____   11._____
5._____   12._____
6._____   13._____
7._____   14._____

PAST HISTORY

Check if you had:

Birth defects_____ Birth injury_____ Feeding problems_____

List all major illnesses and date (or age) when they occurred.

_____   _____   _____

_____   _____   _____

_____   _____   _____

_____   _____   _____

Did you ever smoke?_____ What/how much?_____
Do you smoke now?_____ What/how much?_____

IMMUNIZATION HISTORY

Have you ever had any of the following vaccinations?
Smallpox_____ Date____/____/____
Mumps_____ Date____/____/____
DPT or Tetanus Toxoid_____ Date____/____/____
Measles_____ Date____/____/____
Polio_____ Date____/____/____

COMMUNICABLE DISEASES

Check diseases you have had:
Hepatitis___ Mononucleosis___ Influenza___ Shingles___
Herpes Simplex (cold sores)___ Measles___ German Measles___
Mumps___ Chicken Pox___ Whooping Cough___ Diphtheria___
Scarlet Fever or Scarlatina___ Polio___ Meningitis___
Tuberculosis___ AIDS___ Syphilis___ Gonorrhea___
Other_____

ENDOCRINE

Do you have, or have you ever had, any of the following?
Weight loss of more than five pounds in the past 12 months_____
Weight gain of more than five pounds in the past 12 months_____
Lack of appetite_____ Notable increase in appetite_____
Abnormal thirst_____ Diabetes or sugar in the urine_____
Enlarged thyroid, goiter, over- or under-active thyroid_____
Hypoglycemia_____ Swelling_____ If yes, location_____
Cramps in legs_____

SURGICAL HISTORY

Check if you have had any of the following surgeries, note year performed.

Eye_____   Tonsillectomy_____   Sinus_____
Mastoid_____   Ear_____   Heart_____
Lung_____   Stomach_____   Gallbladder_____
Appendectomy_____   Colon_____   Prostate_____
Brain_____   Bone_____   Skin_____
Cancer_____   Hernia_____   Hemorrhoid_____
Female_____   Other_____   _____

HOSPITALIZATIONS

List reason, length of stay, and dates:

_____
_____
_____
_____
_____

List medical emergencies that required treatment and dates:

_____
_____
_____

Have you had X rays of any of the following? List dates.

Skull_____   Stomach_____   Colon_____
Sinuses_____   Chest_____   Gallbladder_____
Spine_____   Kidneys_____   Extremities_____
Other_____   _____   _____

Have you had any of the following? List dates.

CAT Scan_____   Brain Scan_____
Thyroid Scan_____   Bone Scan_____
EKG _____ Result_____
Stress EKG _____ Result_____
Other_____

FAMILY HISTORY

Check any of the following which have occurred in your family:

Hayfever_____	Hives_____	Constipation_____
Migraine_____	Eczema_____	High Blood
Vertigo_____	Insect Allergy_____	Pressure_____
Asthma_____	Indigestion_____	Low Blood
Emphysema_____	Diarrhea_____	Pressure_____
Arthritis_____	Diabetes_____	Nervousness_____
Heart Diease_____	Stroke_____	Depression_____
Kidney Disease____	Insanity_____	Schizophrenia_____
Epilepsy_____	Drug Use_____	Psychiatric care____
Alcoholism_____	Hypoglycemia_____	Tuberculosis_____
		Drug Allergy_____

FAMILY INFORMATION

Father
If living—Age_____ General Health_____
If deceased—Age at death_____ Cause of death_____

Mother
If living—Age_____ General Health_____
If deceased—Age at death_____ Cause of death_____

Sisters/Brothers
Please note if brother or sister.
#1—_____ If living—Age_____General Health_____
If deceased—Age at death_____ Cause of death_____
#2—_____ If living—Age_____General Health_____
If deceased—Age at death_____ Cause of death_____
#3—_____ If living—Age_____General Health_____
If deceased—Age at death_____ Cause of death_____
#4—_____ If living—Age_____General Health_____
If deceased—Age at death_____ Cause of death_____

Husband/Wife
If living—Age_____ General Health_____
If deceased—Age at death_____ Cause of death_____

Son(s)/Daughter(s)
Please note if son or daughter
#1—_____ If living—Age_____General Health_____
If deceased—Age at death_____ Cause of death_____
#2—_____ If living—Age_____General Health_____
If deceased—Age at death_____ Cause of death_____
#3—_____ If living—Age_____General Health_____
If deceased—Age at death_____ Cause of death_____
#4—_____ If living—Age_____General Health_____
If deceased—Age at death_____ Cause of death_____

Please check any of the following that you have experienced:

Anaphylaxis	____	Emphysema	____	Laryngeal Edema	
Arthritis	____	Diabetes	____		____
Shock	____	Paralysis	____	Psychiatric Care	
Stroke	____	Severe Dizzy			____
Pneumonia	____	Spells	____	Loss of conscious-	
Peptic Ulcer	____	High Blood		ness	____
Convulsions	____	Pressure	____	Tuberculosis	____
Heart Attack	____				

Severe reactions to allergy test or injections_____

EYES

Check any of the following that you have experienced:

Itching	_____	Blurred vision	_____	Crusty lids	_____
Sties	_____	Granulated lids		Cataracts	_____
Irritated	_____		_____	Bloodshot	_____
Watering	_____	Glaucoma	_____	Swelling of	
Dryness	_____	Mucus in eyes	_____	lids	_____
Burning	_____	Puffy under		Twitching of	
Dark circles	_____	eyes	_____	lids	_____
Wear glasses	_____	Wear contacts	_____	Frequent blinking	
Pain	_____	Sensitive to			_____
"Floaters"	_____	light	_____		

Are these problems present all year?_____ If not, in which season are they most common?_____

EARS

Check any of the following that you have experienced:

Hearing loss	_____	Drainage	_____	Frequent	
Dizziness	_____	Loss of		infections	_____
Ever lanced	_____	balance	_____	Fluid accumu-	
Pressure	_____	Itching inside	_____	lation	_____
Pain	_____	Crusting inside	_____	Eustachian block	_____
Ringing	_____	Roaring	_____	Wear hearing	
Nerve		"Floating"		aid	_____
deafness	_____	sensation	_____	Tubes in ears	_____
Other_____					

Are these problems present all year?_____ If not, in which season are they most common?_____

NOSE

Check any of the following that you have experienced:

Itching _____	Post nasal	Require nose
Crusting _____	drip _____	drops _____
Bleeding _____	Blockage _____	Mucus blood-
Dripping _____	Burns _____	streaked _____
Polyps _____	Sneezing _____	Mucus yellow _____
Sinus infections _____	No sense of	Blisters _____
	smell _____	

Other_____

Are these problems present all year?_____ If not, in which season are they most common?_____
More common upon arising_____ after meals_____
after medication_____ lying down_____ at night_____
cold weather_____ hot weather_____ humid weather_____
dry weather_____ other_____

MOUTH AND THROAT

Check any of the following that you have experienced:

Snoring _____	Metallic taste	_____
Hoarse _____	Coated tongue	_____
Lips swell _____	Postnasal drip	_____
Gag easily _____	Grind teeth	_____
Sore throat _____	Sleep with mouth open	_____
Voice loss _____	Lips crack at corners	_____
Bad breath _____	Sore/raw tongue	_____
Bad taste _____	Difficulty swallowing	_____
Dentures _____	Throat/palate itches	_____
Canker sores _____	Throat clearing	_____
Throat closes _____	Neck glands swell	_____
Chapped lips _____	Cracks in tongue	_____
Fever blisters _____	Purplish colored tongue	_____
Tongue swollen _____		

CARDIAC AND RESPIRATORY

Check any of the following that you have experienced:

Wheeze	____	Leg cramps	____
Asthma	____	Chest tightness	____
Murmur	____	Heart attack	____
Croup	____	Chest pains	____
Stroke	____	Shortness of breath	____
Dry cough	____	Frequent infections	____
Angina	____	Night sweats	____
Tingling	____	Swollen ankles	____
Flushing	____	Pneumonia____times	____
Rapid heart	____	Skipped beats	____
Frequent coughs	____	Enlargement	____
Coughing mucus	____	Heaviness in chest	____
Bronchitis	____	Other____	
Frequent colds	____		

How far can you walk vigorously before becoming short of breath?_____

How far can you walk vigorously before leg cramps develop? _____

What is your main problem?_____

When is it worse? morning____ before lunch____ afternoon____ night____ spring____ summer____ fall____ winter____ year round____ other

What, if any, heart medicines are you taking currently?

_____   _____

_____   _____

GASTROINTESTINAL

Check any of the following that you have experienced:

Heartburn	___	Stomach aches	___
Bloating	___	Bloody stools	___
Flatulence	___	Tarry stools	___
Picky eater	___	Frequent nausea	___
Crave sweets	___	Use laxatives	___
Ulcer	___	Anal itching	___
Cramping	___	Roughage intolerance	___
Constipated	___	Belch frequently	___
Diarrhea	___	Fat intolerance	___
Anal pain	___	Gallbladder trouble	___
Vomit blood	___	Frequent vomiting	___
Stool sinks	___	Large bulky stool	___
Indigestion	___	Fragmented stool	___
Retaste food	___	Strong stool odor	___
Good appetite	___	Mucus in stools	___
Poor appetite	___	Light-colored stool	___
Queasy stomach	___	Rectal bleeding	___
Stool floats	___		

MUSCULOSKELETAL

Do you have joint/muscle pain?___ How severe?___
Joint swelling?___ Has fluid been removed?___ When did pain or swelling begin?___ Is it constant or does it vary?___
Do you have morning stiffness?___ How long does it last?___

Were you ever diagnosed with any of the following:

Rheumatoid	___	Multiple sclerosis	___
Lupus	___	Osteoarthritis	___
Rheumatic fever	___	Autoimmune Disease	___
Other	___	Collagen Vascular Disease	___

CONTACT DERMATITIS

Do you have a reaction to contact with any substance?_____
Which substances? _____   _____   _____
Area covered_____ Frequency_____
What treatment has been used?_____
Check if you have ever had: poison oak_____ poison ivy_____
poison sumac_____ other_____
Does metal in contact with your skin cause you to break out?_____

SKIN AND HAIR

Check any of the following that you have experienced:

Eczema	_____	Ringworm	_____
Redness	_____	Oiliness	_____
Itching	_____	Fungus skin	_____
Hives	_____	Burning feet	_____
Rash	_____	Teenage acne	_____
Edema	_____	Excessive loss of hair	_____
Cracking	_____	White spots on nails	_____
Lumps	_____	Brittle nails	_____
Boils	_____	Gooseflesh common	_____
Nodes	_____	Sweating palms	_____
Sores	_____	Cuts heal slowly	_____
Adult acne	_____	Genital herpes	_____
Ridge nails	_____	Foot odors	_____
Scaly lesions	_____	Flush easily	_____
Herpes simplex	_____	Dull hair	_____
Shingles	_____	Athletes foot	_____
Blanching	_____	Bruise easily	_____
Dryness	_____	Peeling	_____
Fungus/nails	_____	Other	_____

List main areas involved._____
Is your skin sensitive to sun_____ fabrics_____ detergents_____
other_____ where_____
frequency_____

INSECT SENSITIVITY

List any insects that cause a more severe reaction than normal.

Check reactions you may have gotten to insect stings or bites:

Hives	_____	Local swelling	_____
Shock	_____	Anaphylaxis	_____
Nausea	_____	Loss of consciousness	_____
Vomiting	_____	Difficulty breathing	_____
Fainting	_____	Difficulty swallowing	_____
Dizziness	_____	Other	_____
Mental confusion	_____	_____	
Required hospitalization	_____	_____	

Do insects seem to single you out?_____
Which insects?_____ _____ _____ _____
How many reactions have you had?_____
What type of treatment do you receive after each reaction?_____
_____

URINARY AND GENITALIA

Check any of the following that you have experienced:

Frequent urination	_____	Genital herpes	_____
Painful urination	_____	Discharge	_____
Difficulty urinating	_____	Pass blood	_____
Lack of control	_____	Sores	_____
Bed-wetting	_____	Trichomonas	_____
Itching	_____	Treated for Trichomonas	_____
Burning	_____	Spouse/Trichomonas	_____
Cystitis	_____	Yeast infections	_____
Kidney disease	_____	Treated for yeast infection	_____
Bladder disease	_____	Cancer	_____
Kidney stones	_____	Location/cancer	_____
Prostate trouble	_____	Impotence	_____
Infection	_____	Frigidity	_____
Treatment for infection	_____	Other	_____

HEADACHE AND CEREBRAL

Check any of the following types of headache pain that you have experienced:

Dull	_____	Constant	_____	Constriction	_____
Sharp	_____	Episodic	_____	Vicelike	_____
Cutting	_____	Throbbing	_____	Pulsating	_____
Boring	_____	Burning	_____	Pressure	_____
Tight	_____	Bandlike	_____	Heaviness	_____
Acute	_____	Caplike	_____	Cramplike	_____
Drawing	_____	Soreness	_____	Excruciating	_____

Check location of pain:

Crown	_____	Back of head	_____
Cheek	_____	Back of neck	_____
Forehead	_____	Lasts minutes	_____
Lasts days	_____	Begins slowly	_____
Back of eye	_____	Right side of head	_____
Lasts hours	_____	Left side of head	_____
Episodic	_____	Returns regularly	_____
Clears completely	_____	Begins suddenly	_____
Top of head	_____	Worse lying down	_____
Upper teeth	_____	Clears w/out treatment	_____
Lasts seconds	_____	Relieved by walking	_____

Check any of the following that are associated with headache:

Nausea	_____	Queasy stomach	_____
Vomiting	_____	Chilly sensation	_____
Pallor	_____	Nasal blockage	_____
Diarrhea	_____	Neck/shoulder pain	_____
Flushing	_____	Visual disturbance	_____
Tearing	_____	Dazzling lights	_____
Running nose	_____	Abdominal pain	_____
Loss of sight	_____	Swelling of eye	_____
Inflamed eye	_____	Other_____	

Check any of the following that precede or intensify pain:

Fear	____	Rejection	____
Anger		Chilling	____
Arguments	____	Fasting	____
Anxiety	____	Motion	____
Eye strain	____	Unusual stimulation	____
Foods	____	Alcoholic drinks	____
Odors	____	Intense thinking	____
Noise	____	Disappointment	____
Exercise	____	Overheating	____
Humidity	____	Infections	____
Intense light	____	Coffee/tea	____
Muscle strain	____	Other_____	

Check when your headache usually occurs:

Spring	____	During sleep	____
Summer	____	On arising	____
Fall	____	Before menstration	____
Winter	____	During menstration	____
On arising	____	After breakfast	____
After lunch	____	When lying down	____
Before supper	____	Before lunch	____
After supper	____		

At what age did headaches begin?_____

Check any of the following that apply when you have a headache·

Can keep working	____	Cannot keep working	____
Require bedrest	____	Require darkness	____
Require eye covering	____	Require hospitalization	____
Pressure to head	____	Hot/cold compresses	____

Check if you have ever had any of the following:

Head injury	____	Back/neck injury	____
Skull fracture	____	Been knocked unconscious	____
Dental occlusion	____	Regular dental care	____
Encephalitis	____		

Check any of the following found in your family history:

Headaches	_____	Undue fatigue	_____
Brain tumors	_____	Emotional Problems	_____
Inhalant allergies	_____	Food allergies	_____
Nervous breakdown	_____	Chemical allergies	_____

Do you know any causes of your headaches?_____ If yes,_____
_____

Has your doctor run any tests?_____ If yes,_____
_____

If you have been hospitalized with a headache, when_____
What treatment did you receive?_____

List medications you take for your headaches:

_____ _____ _____

_____ _____ _____

PSYCHOLOGIC HISTORY

Check any of the following that you have experienced:

Convulsions	_____	Perfectionist	_____
Dizziness	_____	Incessant talker	_____
Fainting	_____	Had nervous breakdown	_____
Blackouts	_____	Family member/nervous	
Amnesia	_____	breakdown	_____
Shock therapy	_____	Use tranquilizers	_____
Hospitalized for		Frequently keyed up/jittery	_____
nerves	_____	Aggressive	_____
Shaky	_____	Startled by sudden noises	_____
Misunderstood by		Often feel suddenly scared	_____
others	_____	Easily get angry	_____
Irritable	_____	Feeling of hostility	_____
Go to pieces easily	_____	Undue fatigue	_____
Forgetful	_____	Pale	_____
Listless	_____	Hyperactive	_____
Stuporous	_____	Feel "lost in time"	_____
Withdrawn feeling	_____	Clumsy	_____
Restless legs	_____	Lack of muscular	
Feel groggy	_____	coordination	_____
Unable to concentrate	_____	Difficulty falling asleep	_____
Short attention span	_____	Difficulty staying asleep	_____
Vision changes	_____	Sleep walking	_____
Unable to reason	_____	Considered a nervous person	_____
State of Anxiety	_____	Worried by little things	_____
Daytime sleepiness	_____	Am a workaholic	_____
Unusual tension	_____	Often unable to	
Frustration	_____	perform work	_____
Numbness	_____	Had hallucinations	_____
Have had visions	_____	Often break out in	
Profuse sweating	_____	cold sweats	_____
Depressed	_____	Heard voices	_____
Cry often	_____	Controlled by other forces	_____
Often unhappy	_____	Seriously considered suicide	_____
Feel insecure	_____	Overused alcohol	_____
Drug addiction	_____	Overused drugs	_____
Concentration	_____	Extremely shy/sensitive	_____
Inner trembling	_____	Other	_____

CHILDREN ONLY

Check any of the following that apply to your child:

Finicky appetite	_____	Whiny/bad tempered	_____
Slow to learn	_____	Intense temper/fury	_____
Clumsy/uncoordinated	_____	Has few friends	_____
Sluggish in morning	_____	Head and neck	
Markedly shy/timid	_____	sweats/sleeping	_____
Hyperactive	_____	Discipline problem	_____
Reading problem	_____	Usually meddlesome	_____
Unable to gain weight	_____	Trouble sleeping	_____
Car sickness	_____	Writing problem	_____
		Other	_____

WOMEN ONLY

Check any of the following that apply to you:

Breast cysts or lumps	_____	Breast soreness	
Breast biopsy	_____	during periods	_____
Mastectomy	_____	Breast soreness	
Breast soreness		unrelated to periods	_____
before periods	_____		

CHILDBIRTH

Number of children_____ Normal Birth(s)_____

Normal Pregnancy_____ If not explain_____

Difficult labor_____ Explain_____

Birthweight(s)_____ _____ _____ Infant(s) normal_____

Miscarriage(s)_____ If so, reason_____

Problems with infant(s)_____

MENSES

Age of onset	____	Scant flow	____
Had D & C	____	Use diaphragm	____
Use IUD	____	Trying to get pregnant	____
Heavy flow	____	Irregular periods	____
Use foam	____	Regular periods	____
Had hysterectomy	____	Use douches	____
Partial	____	Use lubricants	____
Total	____	Other female surgery____	
Miscarriage	____	_____	
Now pregnant	____		

What problems do you have before periods?_____
_____
Duration_____
Problems at ovulation? (Middle of cycle)_____
Duration_____

MENOPAUSE

Age of menopause____ Taking hormones?____ How long?____

FOOD HISTORY

Which of the following have you experienced:

Weight loss	____	Excessive hunger	____
Weight gain	____	Excessive thirst	____
Crave beverages	____	Overindulge foods	____
Crave certain foods	____	Dislike certain foods	____
Avoid certain foods	____	Bothered by food odors	____
Eat junk food	____	Eat daytime snacks	____
Skip meals	____	Have bedtime snacks	____
Crash diets	____	Eat regular meals	____
Elimination diets	____	Rotation diets	____
Caveman diets	____	Use convenience foods	____
Cook from "scratch"	____	Use exotic foods	____
Other____		_____	

Have you ever been on a special diet?____
List_____
Crave or dislike certain foods?____
List_____

As an infant did you have any of the following:

Colic	____	Skin rash	____	Bothered by foods	____
Eczema	____	Headaches	____	Learning problem	____
Hives	____	Bed-wetting	____	Failure to thrive	____
Diarrhea	____	Poor appetite	____	Constant hunger	____
Gassiness	____	Night sweats	____	Stomach aches	____
Dyslexia	____	Picky eater	____	Recurrent infection	____
Bottle fed	____	Constipation	____	Ear infections	____
Vomiting	____	Hyperactivity	____	Behavior problem	____
Leg aches	____	Fussiness	____		

Other_____

What happens if you miss a meal?_____
Is there a family history of allergies or food intolerance?____
Do you eat most of your meals: at home____ restaurants____
gourmet meals____
Do you mainly eat foods that are: fresh____ canned____
frozen____ prepackaged____

FOOD LIST

On the following list of foods please use the letter to describe
your feelings about each one.

A   Eat daily
B   Eat few times a week
C   Eat seldom
D   Never eat
E   Crave/really like
F   Don't like
G   Like but bothers me
H   Like, but avoid or limit

Allspice	_____	Caraway	_____	Curry	_____
Almond	_____	Carob	_____	Dates	_____
Apple	_____	Carrot	_____	Dill	_____
Apricot	_____	Cashew	_____	Duck	_____
Arrowroot	_____	Celery	_____	Egg	_____
Artichoke	_____	Cheddar cheese	_____	Eggplant	_____
Asparagus	_____	Cherry	_____	Endive	_____
Avocado	_____	Chewing gum	_____	Fig	_____
Banana	_____	Chicken	_____	Flounder	_____
Barley	_____	Chicory	_____	Fish/Sea	
Basil	_____	Chili pepper	_____	Cod	_____
Bay Leaf	_____	Chili powder	_____	Halibut	_____
Kidney beans	_____	Chocolate	_____	Perch	_____
Lima beans	_____	Cocoa	_____	Red Snapper	_____
Navy beans	_____	Cinnamon	_____	Sole	_____
Pinto beans	_____	Citrus juice	_____	Fish, fresh	_____
Beef	_____	Grapefruit	_____	Bass	_____
Beets	_____	Lemon	_____	Catfish	_____
Bell pepper	_____	Lime	_____	Perch	_____
Blackberry	_____	Orange	_____	Salmon	_____
Blueberry	_____	Clam	_____	Sturgeon	_____
Raspberry	_____	Clove	_____	Trout	_____
Black-eyed peas	_____	Coconut oil	_____	Garlic	_____
Brazil Nut	_____	Coffee	_____	Gelatin	_____
Buckwheat	_____	Cola	_____	Ginger	_____
Cabbage	_____	Cottage cheese	_____	Grapes	_____
Broccoli	_____	Crab	_____	Haddock	_____
Brussel sprout	_____	Cranberry	_____	Hazelnut	_____
Cauliflower	_____	Cucumber	_____	Honey	_____

Hops ___	Oregano ___	Saccharin ___
Horseradish ___	Orris root ___	Safflower oil ___
Herring ___	Oyster ___	Sage ___
Karaya gum ___	Papaya ___	Salt ___
Lamb ___	Paprika ___	Sardine ___
Lentil ___	Parmesan	Scallop ___
Lettuce ___	cheese ___	Sesame seed
Licorice ___	Parsley ___	oil ___
Lobster ___	Parsnip ___	Shrimp ___
Mackerel ___	Peas ___	Soy ___
Tangerine ___	Peach ___	Spinach ___
Mango ___	Peanut oil ___	Squash ___
Maple syrup ___	Pear ___	Strawberry ___
Cantaloupe ___	Pecan ___	String bean ___
Casaba melon ___	Pepper ___	Sugar beet ___
Honeydew	Pimento ___	Sugar cane ___
melon ___	Pineapple ___	Sunflower seed ___
Persian melon ___	Pistachio ___	Swiss cheese ___
Milk, cow ___	Plum ___	Tapioca ___
Milk, goat ___	Poppy seed ___	Tea ___
Peppermint ___	Pork ___	Thyme ___
Spearmint ___	Potato, sweet ___	Tomato ___
Molasses ___	Potato, white ___	Tuna ___
Mung bean ___	Prune ___	Turkey ___
Mushrooms ___	Pumpkin seeds ___	Turnip ___
Mustard ___	Rabbit ___	Vanilla ___
Mustard green ___	Radish ___	Venison ___
Nutmeg ___	Raisins ___	Walnut,
Oats ___	Rhubarb ___	English ___
Okra ___	Rice ___	Watermelon ___
Olive oil ___	Roquefort ___	Wheat ___
Onion ___	Rye ___	Yeast ___

Pie, fruit ___	Pie, cream ___	Potato chips ___
Cakes ___	Cookies ___	Candy ___
Corn chips ___	Mayonnaise ___	Ketchup ___
Ice cream ___	Prepared dinners ___	Yogurt ___
Jams/jelly ___	Processed foods ___	

NUTRITIONAL HISTORY

Please list the foods you normally consume on a daily basis.
Include snacks, beverages, and so forth.

Breakfast:_____
_____
_____
_____

Lunch:_____
_____
_____
_____

Dinner:_____
_____
_____
_____

Snacks:_____
_____
_____

Supplements taken:_____
_____
_____

Other:_____
_____

ALLERGY TREATMENT

Have you ever had allergy tests:_____
When:_____ Where:_____ What type:_____
Physician's name:_____ Are you taking allergy
injections or medication now?_____ What type:_____
Have you ever required adrenalin injects for allergy?_____
How many times?_____ Have you ever required emergency
treatment for an allergic reaction?_____ How many times?_____
Other:_____

INHALANT AND CHEMICAL HISTORY

Occupational Information:

Teacher	_____	Work around fumes	_____
Painter	_____	Work with animals	_____
Salesperson	_____	Professional	_____
Farm work	_____	Work around dust	_____
Housework	_____	Hospital work	_____
Work outdoors	_____	Work around cosmetics	_____
Office work	_____	Work in extreme heat	_____
Factory work	_____	Work in extreme cold	_____
Construction work	_____	Other_____	
Work indoors	_____	_____	

Do you feel better at work?_____ Worse?_____ Same?_____

Check any of the following that cause irritation:

Dust	_____	Chemicals	_____	Central heat/cool	_____
Mildew	_____	Grain dust	_____	Artist's supplies	_____
Molds	_____	Fireplace	_____	Fresh newspapers	_____
Slab home	_____	Potted plants	_____	Old magazines	_____
New home	_____	Tobacco smoke	_____	Photocopy paper	_____
Old home	_____	Disinfectants	_____	Gas stove/heat	_____
Feathers	_____	Old carpet	_____	Furniture polish	_____
Rugs	_____	New carpet	_____	Space heaters	_____
Cotton	_____	Solvents	_____	Floor furnace	_____
Kapok	_____	Cosmetics	_____	Diesel fuel	_____
Sisal	_____	Eye makeup	_____	Detergents	_____
Hemp	_____	Nail polish	_____	Exhaust fumes	_____
Glue	_____	Marshy areas	_____	Wooded areas	_____
Tar	_____	Wood smoke	_____	Gasoline fumes	_____
Soaps	_____	Deodorants	_____	Perfumes	_____
Paints	_____	Drapes	_____	Bird inside	_____
Dog inside	_____	Cat inside	_____	Other pet inside	_____
Rubber	_____	Raised home	_____	Insecticides	_____
Dyes	_____	Floor wax	_____	Turpentine	_____
Alcohol	_____	Hairsprays	_____	Overstuffed	
Plastic	_____	Herbicides	_____	furniture	_____
Incense	_____	Mothballs	_____	Fertilizers	_____
Newsprint	_____	Varnishes	_____	Lacquers	_____

Check if you have reactions in the following conditions:

Spring	_____	In moldy areas	_____
Summer	_____	Raking leaves	_____
Fall	_____	Certain localities	_____
Winter	_____	Physically exerted	_____
Year long	_____	When cutting grass	_____
Certain rooms	_____	Humid/windy weather	_____
Housecleaning	_____	Worse at night	_____
Specific odors	_____		

List family hobbies:_____

_____

List family exposures:_____

_____

Note brand name of any of the following products you use regularly:

Tobacco_____	Cough drops_____	Laundry detergent_____
Soap_____	Chewing gum_____	Fabric softener_____
Shampoo_____	Dentifrice_____	After-shave_____
Perfume_____	Chapstick_____	Dental adhesive_____
Lipstick_____	Toothpaste_____	Mouthwash_____

ENVIRONMENT

Do you live in an apartment?_____ How old?_____
Do you live in a house?_____ How old?_____
Other housing_____
Does your home tend to get dustier than other homes?_____
Does your home seem to be drier than other homes?_____
Does your home seem to be damper than other homes?_____
Does it have a basement?_____ Have you ever noticed mold or mildew in your home?_____

HEATING SYSTEM

Gas furnace	_____	Floor furnace	_____
Oven	_____	Electric baseboard	_____
Stove	_____	Electric panel	_____
Fireplace	_____	Radiator steam heat	_____
Oil furnace	_____	Space heater	_____
Wall furnace	_____	Other_____	
Hot water heat	_____		

PILLOW

Your pillow consists of:
Feather _____   Kapok   _____   Synthetic _____
Down _____   Foam rubber_____   Other_____

Roommate's pillow:
Feather _____   Kapok   _____   Synthetic _____
Down _____   Foam rubber _____   Other_____

MATTRESS

Water bed_____ Conventional_____ Box spring/interspring_____
Foam rubber_____ Other_____

BLANKETS

Wool_____ Cotton_____ Quilt_____ Synthetic_____
Other_____

ANIMALS/PETS

Dog   _____   Cat   _____   Rabbits   _____
Birds   _____   Horses _____   Hamsters _____
Guinea pig _____   Cattle   _____   Other_____

PLANTS

Do you have indoor plants?_____ Number_____

DRUG/MEDICATION HISTORY

Check medications taken regularly:

Aspirin	_____	Food supplements	_____
Iron	_____	Laxatives	_____
Codeine	_____	Vitamins	_____
Insulin	_____	Mycin drugs	_____
Demerol	_____	Blood pressure medicine	_____
Hormones	_____	Phenobarbital	_____
Minerals	_____	Birth control pills	_____
Nose drops	_____	Rx medications	_____
Dilantin	_____	Penicillin	_____
Antibiotics	_____	Tranquilizers	_____
Tylenol	_____	Sleeping pills	_____
Cortisone	_____	Sulfa drugs	_____
Digitalis	_____	Antihistimines	_____
Cough medicine	_____	Other_____	
Paregoric	_____	_____	
Adrenalin	_____		

List any drugs or medication which cause a reaction:

_____ _____ _____

_____ _____ _____

Have you ever reacted to:

Dental anesthetics	_____	Tetanus antitoxin	_____
Tetanus toxoid	_____	X-ray contrast media	_____
Iodides	_____		

Do you require adjusted doses of medication:_____

Instructions for Taking Blood Pressure

Place the cuff on the left arm with the stethoscope part of the cuff at the bottom. The cuff should rest just above the bend of your elbow with the stethoscope toward the inside of your arm. You should be able to bend your arm and have the bottom of the cuff rest in the crook of your arm. Pull the cuff until it is snug (you should be able to insert two fingers under the cuff before it is inflated), secure in place by wrapping the cuff around your arm and hooking the Velcro closing. Place the earpieces in your ears.

Your left arm should be resting comfortably on your lap or on a low surface, and should be totally relaxed. If your arm is tense or your fist is clenched, the reading is quite different and not accurate.

Pick up the bulb in your right hand and place the valve between your thumb and index finger. Practice tightening and releasing the valve.

Slowly inflate the cuff with the valve closed (turn clockwise to tighten). Inflate the cuff until the needle reaches 100, listen for sounds. Continue inflating the cuff until you no longer hear any heart sounds, do this slowly, just a little at a time. Pump it up **only to a point where you do not hear any sounds**. It could be painful if you inflate the cuff too far above the point that is necessary.

Slowly release the valve until the needle falls slowly and moves at each heart sound. When you hear the first sound, this is the **systolic**, or upper number of your blood pressure.

Continue releasing the pressure so the needle falls slowly and steadily. If the needle stops and stays in one place, release the valve a little more and it will start to fall again.

The last number on the dial, when you can hear your heart sounds, is the bottom number of your blood pressure, the **diastolic**.

Write down the number when you first heard heart sounds, systolic, and the last, diastolic. This is your blood pressure. *Example:* If you heard your heart sounds at 125 for the first time and the last was at 60, your blood pressure would be written, 125/60.

Practice taking your blood pressure and that of others. You will be surprised at how fast you will learn to listen for the different sounds and intensity.

Recording the Heart Sounds

The Life Balances Health Program requires a much more detailed explanation of a patient's blood pressure. For our records, it is important to note the various sounds of each heartbeat and where it appears on the number line (see enclosed sheets).

We use a series of circles or dots to denote the type of heart sound.

A *loud sound* is a large circle, a *soft sound* is a small dot. Each mark should appear on the number line as you hear it when taking the patient's blood pressure.

Example: If a patient has a blood pressure of 140/80 we would write it out in the standard form on the check sheet first. Then transpose it to a number line, including the different sounds.

$$\underset{\displaystyle 140 \qquad\qquad 120 \qquad\qquad\qquad 90 \qquad\qquad 80}{\circ\circ\circ\circ\circ\bigcirc\bigcirc\bigcirc\bigcirc\bigcirc\bigcirc\bigcirc\circ\circ\circ\circ}$$

If the heart sound came in soft at 140 and got stronger at 120, the circles would be larger at 120, if they were strong until 90, then got softer and quit at 80, the circles would appear as they do in the above example.

If an individual's heart sounds are sloshy or have a pronounced *shhh* sound, then a slash through the circle (0) at the appropriate number would represent this sound.

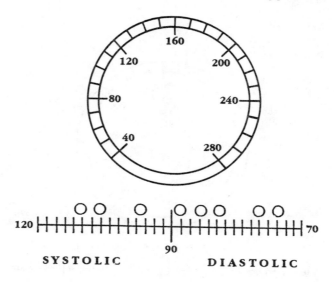

Here is an example of a person's blood pressure. This person has a low fluid level and has an erratic heartbeat. The Life Balances Health Program uses these diagrams to accurately interpret the blood pressure information.

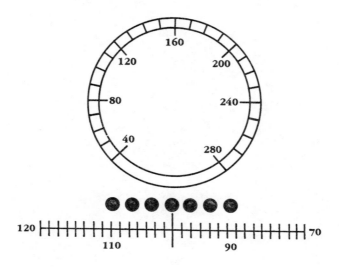

This person has a blood pressure of 110/90. The heart sounds come in solid and go out solid.

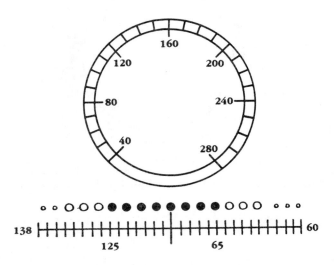

This patient's blood pressure comes in faint at 138, then gets strong at 125 and starts to fade at 65 and is gone at 60.

Bibliography

Barnes, Broda, and Galton. *Hypothyroidism: The Unsuspected Illness*. New York: Thomas Y. Crowell, 1976.

Coca, A. F. *The Pulse Test*. New York: Arco Publishing, 1972.

Cousins, Norman. *Anatomy of an Illness*. New York: W. W. Norton, 1979.

Eaton, S. Boyd, Shostak, M. and Konner, M. *The Paleolithic Prescription*. New York: Harper and Row, 1988.

Eaton, S. Boyd, and Konner, Melvin. "Paleolithic Nutrition." *New England Journal of Medicine, 312:* #5, 31 January 1985, pp. 283–288.

Horrobin, D. F., editor. *Clinical Uses of Essential Fatty Acids*. Montreal: Eden Press, 1982.

Kalokerinos, Archie, M.D. *Every Second Child*. New Canaan, CT: Keats Publishing (paperback), 1981.

Ott, J. N. *Light, Radiation, and You*. Old Greenwich, CT: Devin Adair Co., 1982.

Pauling, Linus, et al. *Orthomolecular Psychiatry*. San Francisco: Freeman Press, 1973.

Price, Weston. *Nutrition and Physical Degeneration*. New Canaan, CT: Keats Publishing, 1989.

Rapp, Doris. *Allergies and the Hyperactive Child*. New York: Cornerstone, 1979.

Schoenthaler, S. J. "The Northern California Diet/Behavior program: An empirical evaluation of 3,000 incarcerated juveniles in

Stanislaus County Juvenile Hall." *International Journal of Biosocial Research*, 5: #2, 1983, pp. 99–106.

Schoenthaler, S. J., Ph.D., Doraz, W., Ph.D., Wakefield, J., Ph.D., "The Impact of a low Food Additive and Sucrose Diet in Academic Performance in 803 New York City Public Schools," *International Journal of Biosocial Research*, Tacoma, WA. 8: #2, 1986, pp. 185–195.

Selye, Hans. *Stress Without Distress*. New York: Lippincott, 1974.

Smith, Lendon H., M.D. *Clinical Guide to the Use of Vitamin C; The Clinical Experiences of Frederick Klenner, M.D.* Tacoma, WA: Life Sciences Press, 1988.

Williams, Roger. *Biochemical Individuality: The Basis for the Genotrophic Concept*. New York: Wiley, 1956.

Index

abdomen, 41
acidity, 12. *See also* pH
acupuncture, 23, 35
acupuncturists, 18
adenoids, 124
aging, 124
AIDS, 73, 205–208
alcoholism, 47, 69, 70, 125
Alzheimer's disease, 184–185
alkalinity, 12, 58–59. *See also* pH
allergies, 67, 68, 201–202, 209. *See also* food sensitivies
allopathic approaches, 19
allopathic doctors, 11; and the pharmaceutical industry, 19, 20, 33, 37
alopecia, 125–128
amenorrhea, 128
American Medical Association, 26
amino acids, 213–220
anemia, 68, 69, 70, 72, 128
anorexia, 67, 68, 69, 70, 128
anthropological studies, 32–35, 42–43, 219
antibiotics, 26–27
anxiety, 67, 174–175
arthritis, 50, 68, 70, 129
asthma, 67, 71, 209
ayurvedic medicine, 23

backache, 129
bad breath, 129
Bates, Dr. Charles, 219
bed-wetting, 16, 17; food sensitivies and, 16, 29, 34–35, 50; nutritional deficiencies and, 29; psychiatric approach to, 16; vitamin therapy for, 35
behavior: aggressive, 184; relationship to diet, 31–32
biochemistry, individual. *See* body chemistry
biotechnology, 28
blood pressure. *See* Hypertension
blood sugar, low, 67, 70, 136
blood tests, 15, 20; and electrolytes, 151;

blood tests *(continued)*:
    a key to nutritional deficiencies, 94;
    how to read, 93–121
Board of Medical Examiners, 33
body chemistry, individual, 12–13, 15, 18, 37, 46, 49, 52; attending to, 65–66; and body fluids, 144–151; and electrolytes, 143–151; normal, 93–112
body type, 15–16, 18
bone spurs, 129
Boussingault, Jean-Baptiste, 79–80
breast: cysts, 41, 130; feeding, 130; tender, 41
bursitis, 130

California Reading Teachers Association, 32
canker sores, 40
cancer, 209–210
cardiac arrhythmia, 130
carpal tunnel syndrome, 41, 67, 130
cataract, 131
Cathcart, Dr. Robert, 50
celiac disease, 131
chemical imbalance. *See* body chemistry
chemical laws, 75–79; and nutrition, 79
chiropractors, 18, 35
chocolate cravings, 57–58
cholesterol, 68, 69, 70, 72, 131
colic, 131–132
colitis, 132
conjunctivitis, 66, 67
constipation, 132
Cousins, Norman, 34
Crohn's disease, 132
cystic fibrosis, 132

dandruff, 39, 49, 66, 67, 132
Davis, Adelle, 49
depression, 52–53, 67, 70, 72, 189
diabetes, 68, 70, 133
diarrhea, 53, 66, 68, 69, 70, 72, 133
diet: changes in history, 42–43;
    hereditary basis for individual, 43;
    in Paleolithic era, 42; relation to

liver cirrhosis of, 131. *See also* alcoholism
lupus, 210

magnesium dependency, 51
Marsh, Dr. Richard, 7
memory loss, 67, 69, 72, 137
Ménière's syndrome, 137
menopause, 137
menstruation, 66, 68
metabolism, 16
migraine, 50, 71, 137–138
Mindell, Earl, 49
Monte, Dr. Woodrow C., 185
mononucleosis, 50
multiple sclerosis, 138
muscle cramps, 68, 138
myopia, 68

nails, finger and toe, 40, 49, 66, 68, 69, 70, 72
Native American cures, 25
naturopathic physicians, 18, 35, 175, 184
neurotransmitters, 180–182
nose, bleeding, 39
numbness, 67, 69, 131
nutrition: and environment, 89–91; and the family, 17; and the immune system, 32; individual program of, 15; limitations of, 35, 49; and topsoil, 89, 91; and senses of smell and taste, 20, 60–63, 65–74; and traditional medicine, 16
nutritional dependencies, 52
nutritionists, 18

obesity, 138
odors, body, 138
osteoporosis, 68, 138–139

Palmer, David D., 25
Paracelsus, 24
paranoia, 67, 70
parasites, 139
Passwater, Richard, 49
Pasteur, Louis, 25
Pauling, Linus, 49, 90
perfect health, 45–46
persperation, excessive, 39
pH, 114, 118, 144; testing, 59–60
pharmaceuticals: and hypertension, 159–160; reliance of doctors upon, 19, 28

pneumonia, viral, 50
polyps, 39
pregnancy, 139
prementrual syndrome (PMS), 67, 68, 139
prostate hypertrophy, 139
psoriasis, 139–140
predispositions. *See* genetics
Price, Dr. Weston, 42–43
Priessnitz, 25

RDA, 52, 80; limitations of, 81–88
Ringer, Dr. Sidney, 148–149, 155–156
Ritalin, 30, 193, 222, 227

Sackler, Dr. Arthur, 88
schizphrenia, 180–184
Schoenthaler, Stephen, 30–31
Selye, Hans, 203–205
Seattle, Chief, 233
skin problems: acne, 39, 49, 66, 72, 124; dermatitis, 67; on arms, 40; on hands, 40–41; behind ears, 39; around eyes, 39, 66; on feet, 41; on neck, 40; pallor, 39, 67; of the scalp, 39. *See also* eczema
slipped disc, 140
stomachaches, 140
stressors, to the body, 46, 50
stroke, 140
Sudden Infant Death Syndrome (SIDS), 27, 32
surgical techniques: developing proficiency of, 19–20

tongue problems, 40, 68, 69, 70
tooth decay, 68, 69
Typhoid Mary, 26

ulcers, 140

varicose veins, 41
vision problems, 140–141
vitamin and mineral deficiencies, 51–52; as shown by blood tests, 94–112; BCl (Betaine Hydrocloride), 69; biotin, 68; calcium, 69, 119; chlorine, 68–69; chromium, 72; copper, 72; folic acid, 69; iron, 69–70; magnesium, 57–58, 70, 120–121; manganese, 72; NH,Cl (Ammonium Chloride), 71; Paraminobenzoic Acid, 70; Panthothenic Acid, 70–71; potassium, 71, 119–120;

vitamin and mineral deficiencies
(continued) :
    sodium, 119; vitamin A, 49, 66; vitamin
B₁, 66–67; vitamin B₂, 67; vitamin B₃,
70; vitamin B₆, 67; vitamin B₁₂, 67;
vitamin C, 67–68; vitamin D, 68;
vitamin E, 68; zinc, 72
vitamin therapies: for ankylosing
    spondylitis, 34; for hyperactivity,
29–32; for flu symptoms, 54–55;
individual daily, 61–63; intravenous,
50–51, 53; for memory problems, 55;

vitamin therapies *(continued)* :
    as a routine treatment for pathologies,
33–34, 39–41, 50–51; for SIDS, 32.
See also Life Balances Health Program

Walsh, Dr. William, 184
warts, 41, 49, 54, 66, 141
Williams, Dr. Roger, 37, 49, 52, 66

x-rays, in medical history, 27
yeast infection, 210